A Nurse's Tales: From Drama to Trauma

Stories of Lynda Johnson, RN

Written by Everett Escobar

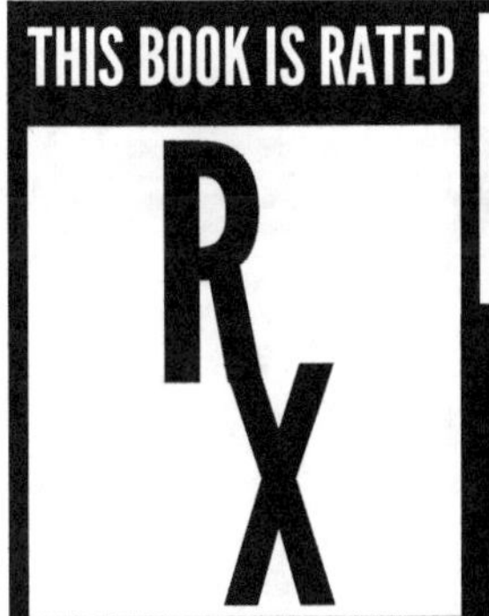

Edited by Everett Escobar & Aerias Hurd
Written by Everett Escobar
Illustrations by Everett Escobar

1st Edition 2024

Foreword

In **_'A Nurse's Tales: From Drama to Trauma,_** _'_ we take a poignant look into the life of Nurse Lynda Johnson, who has been engaged in the nursing field since the age of seventeen. Nurse Johnson's life has spanned over eight decades, and despite any personal ups and downs, she has selflessly touched countless lives and rendered service to others through her compassion, knowledge, and skillset in the nursing field.

It has been an honor for our team to listen to these tales first-hand and encapsulate them within this work. As you read the following pages, I hope you feel the heart and dedication that our Honored Abilities Team has placed into producing this work of historical significance. Most importantly, I hope you can hear Lynda's voice in the tales she's lived to tell.

We hope this publication accurately educates its readers on the drama and trauma that nurses see and endure. May all who read this book gain a greater appreciation for all nurses. This work is dedicated to them for their ever-endearing sacrifices and selfless actions for society as a whole. They truly are the backbone of the healthcare industry. In conjunction with Lynda's Tales, there is also a resource that provides both first aid and nursing tips.

Thank you to all the nurses,

Aerias Hurd, President of Honored Abilities

A Letter From The Nurse

Life has been a treasure for me. I have seen much transpire throughout this world, including turbulent politics, military uprisings, the great awakening of modern technology, civil unrest, economic volatility, and the progression of the ethical workplace.

Though this work is considered a memoir, I intended for the primary focus to be something other than my life story. Instead, I share my stories and a few experiences from others to showcase society's transformation and the obstacles that women in the workplace face, specifically in the healthcare industry.

Though specific names have been changed to safeguard anonymity, every event detailed in this collective work is true and will undoubtedly strike a variety of emotions within you. This work aims to bring a greater understanding and appreciation for current and former nurses everywhere. It has been very apparent to me that most individuals have no idea what nurses have endured daily throughout their careers throughout the decades.

I would like to thank my family for the sacrifices they made during my career. I would also like to thank Lou Trotti, who has lent her nursing knowledge and experiences to see this work through. Lastly, I would especially like to thank *Honored Abilities* for bringing these tales to life in a thought-provoking and captivating manner. I could not have done this without you.

Thank you, and enjoy,

Lynda Johnson

Lynda Johnson, R.N.

The Heart to Start

I was blessed to start nursing school in the late 1950s, particularly in Houston because it allowed me to witness greatness and learn skills and techniques from two of the world's most outstanding heart surgeons. Their friendly rivalry pushed them to test what was considered impossible. These surgeons would eventually be coined 'The Fathers of Modern Cardiovascular Surgery.'

These doctors contributed to developing the artificial heart and many other devices that revolutionized heart surgery. In their field, they were esteemed celebrities. Everyone knew about them and their long list of accolades and accomplishments. They were world-renowned and traveled the world, showcasing their discoveries and techniques to other health professionals. Both were viewed and treated as gods.

I was fortunate to study this field at the same hospital as these doctors as they continued making more wonderful discoveries in cardiology. It was an exciting experience as I constantly saw people worldwide come to them for treatment. Though many of their treatments and procedures were still considered experimental and potentially life-threatening, they had won the confidence of the people who felt that these two surgeons were their best hope for survival, so most volunteered to take the chance.

As students, we would observe dozens of others as they performed various surgeries. It wasn't uncommon for many of these patients to die shortly after surgery, but their deaths were not in vain as it allowed these surgeons to perfect their processes, which allowed for countless lives to be saved in the future.

Each one of their patients had a private on-duty nurse to

The Heart to Start (continued)

watch over them after these delicate procedures. I remember a foreign man that came across the operating table. To resolve his issue, he received a foot-long graft along his femoral artery. Following his surgery, he was tasked with a couple of weeks of rest before engaging in the process of being discharged.

As he packed his belongings to return home, his graft blew, causing all of his blood to rush out all at once. He died instantaneously. Over time, we realized that it would take at least two months of hospital rest for a graft of that size to take, not a couple of weeks. Yet again, these procedures were experimental, so not everyone made it home alive, but to these patients, the potential outcome was worth the risk.

It was fun to be a student at this hospital and to see so many remarkable things unfold and come to fruition. During my last month of school, the first ICU was established at this facility. This allowed us to learn and understand how an ICU worked prior to graduating. It was amazing to be on the cutting edge and to be present when a lot of innovations first started.

I was only disappointed that I wasn't able to witness these two surgeons carry out the first human heart transplant conducted in the United States, which took place in 1968, several years after I graduated from nursing school.

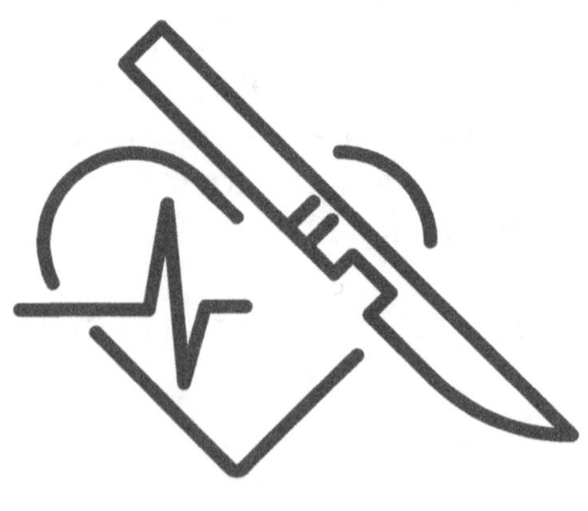

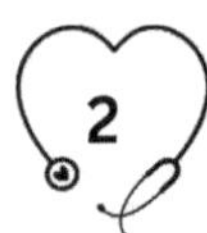

Fallopian Tubes

During my time in nursing school, there were a variety of local outbreaks consisting of polio, diphtheria, typhoid fever, whooping cough, red measles, German measles, chicken pox, and scarlet fever. I often circulated in surgery with a regular nurse in my nursing program. One day, while in the operating room with my other fellow students, our instructor surgeon turned to me and directed, "Student, go get me some fallopian tubes." As a student nurse, if the doctor instructs you to do something, you do it. So, I immediately sprang into action in a desperate search for these fallopian tubes.

Instinctively, I ran to central supply because most of our supplies could be found there. As I frantically rummaged through the room, another person kindly asked, "What are you looking for?" I urgently gasped, "Fallopian tubes! I need to find them and take them to surgery." After a moment, she empathetically replied, "Well, I'm sorry, but we don't have those. The woman has them."

Her statement caught me by surprise and caused me to turn about to face her. Carrying a fixed, shocked expression, I concernedly asked, "What woman?" At this point, I could tell this person was shocked as she stared back at me. After briefly hesitating to respond, she said, "They're already in the woman you're operating on. There's no need to go around searching for them."

I was so confused and dumbfounded. When I arrived back in the operating room, the doctor asked me if I had brought the fallopian tubes that he'd requested. I was nervous and didn't know how to proceed with the conversation. With some hesitation, I pointed to the operating table and replied, "Well, I was told they are in that woman."

With an intrigued expression and a raised brow, the surgeon

Fallopian Tubes (continued)

inquired, "So, you're telling me that the fallopian tubes are in this woman that lays on my operating table?" I swiftly gave an anxious gulp and said, "Yes, sir. They are. At least that's what central supply told me." The doctor folded his arms, cocked his head to the side, and asked, "Do you think central supply knows more than me? A surgeon."

Oh, gosh! This was dreadful. I didn't mean to question his intelligence. I was merely relaying the information that I'd been given. I was frozen and stood there, not knowing what to do. The entire operating room was eerily quiet as I had my verbal exchange with our instructor. Behind me, I could hear soft, subtle whispers taking place. Undoubtedly, their remarks were directed towards me. Ugh! I felt so embarrassed.

What was I going to do? There needed to be a better response to his question. I couldn't bear the awkward silence any longer, so I was quick to sheepishly utter, "I guess so..." As a result, the whole room erupted in a symphony of laughter, and the surgeon gasped in laughter, "You've got to be kidding me!"

Everyone was hooting and hollering—everyone except me and the patient, of course. I was certain that I turned a flush beet red. I was on the receiving end of this big joke. I was so ignorant and gullible then. Thankfully, I did find the joke somewhat humorous myself. As my time in the nursing program went on, I realized that all of our instructors would routinely try to pull jokes on us students.

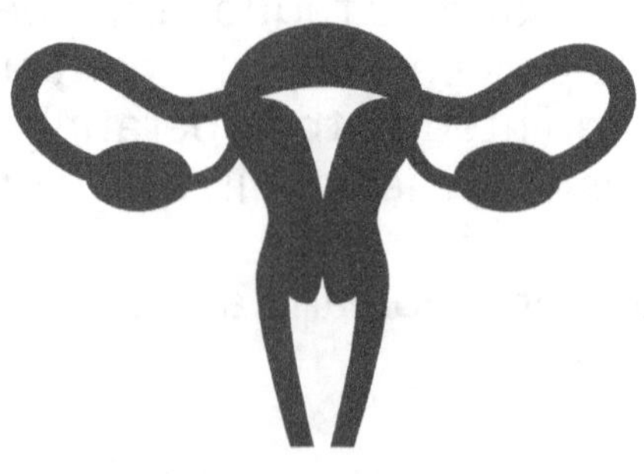

The Gag Affair

As students, we often had to try practices and concepts on each other. One of the things we had to experience was using a Miller-Abbott tube. If you didn't know, they are very long—over nine feet of tubing! At one end of the tube, you find a mercury tip. The Miller-Abbott tube was used to decompress and treat obstructions to the small intestine.

To gain such an experience, we each had to swallow the tube to start the intubation process. Once I had my tube in place, I rolled up the remaining eight feet and pinned it to my clothing.

We were required to wear it all day long. The tube made our typical actions awkward and uncomfortable. The farther into our day we got, the more miserable we became because the tube would slowly work its way farther into our intestines. Our instructors felt that we'd learn better if we conducted this process on ourselves.

It wasn't enjoyable! Breathing, talking, sneezing, belching, passing gas, and even having a bowel movement was tedious. And you could only hope that you had a bowel movement before the tube had found its exit point; otherwise, there would be more you'd have to do besides wiping yourself.

What was also unfortunate was that we had to patiently allow the entire tube length to pass through our system. I wish I could tell you this was the only time we had to intubate ourselves, but sadly it wasn't. During my senior year, I had to experience a Levin tube.

Levin tubes are used for gastric suction, irrigation, and administering medication. We each were put with a fellow student partner who would push the tube through our

The Gag Affair (continued)

nostril and down our throats.

Due to recently having my appendix removed and already having experienced the Miller-Abbott tube, I begged and pleaded to get out of being intubated. My pleas and requests were denied, and I was forced to face another grueling, miserable act.

Paired with my partner, I could feel that my impending doom was near. I remained content and relaxed until she got the tube in my lung, causing me to cough and gag uncontrollably. As I wiped away my tears and readied myself for another attempt, I could hear our instructors correcting my partner and urging her to start again.

I couldn't help but keep my eyes closed. Why did I have to allow myself to be tortured again? It felt very inhumane. Thankfully, she took our instructor's counsel well and correctly set the tube. Even after she had completed the action, I still had a residual cough and sniffles.

I then took some time to breathe and collect myself before carrying out the action on her. My dark inner conscious wanted so badly to mess with her tube so that she'd feel similarly to me, but I knew that if I did that, she'd think that it was a retaliatory act. With great focus and caution, I inserted and guided a portion of the Levin tube down her throat.

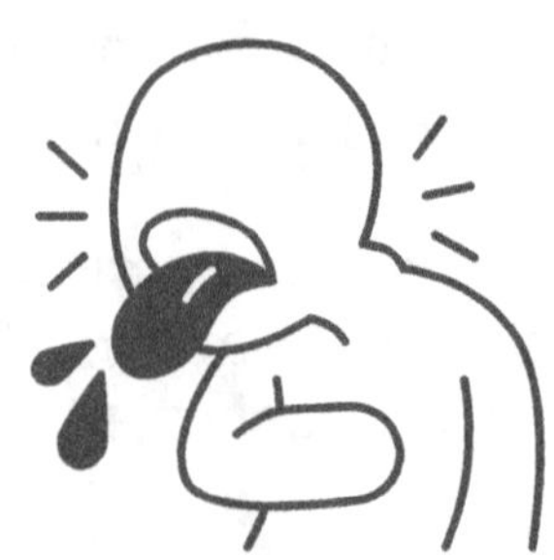

A Little Salty

While I was still a student nurse, I was assigned a patient with a kidney disease called Uremia. One day, I came to visit her and noticed that her arms were incredibly white. Upon further examination, I realized that her arms were rough and crusty. I could tell that she wasn't very comfortable. Just a simple touch of her arm would cause thick, white granules to come off.

Confused by what I had seen, I left the room and spoke with a mentor who explained that the patient's urine was manifesting this way. The urine was coming out as salt from the body. As soon as you wiped it off, the salt granules would return.

Sadly, in her current state and age, there was not much that we could do for my patient. All I could do was help her be more comfortable. However, over time, the rest of her body began showcasing this salty symptom, and she eventually died from her condition.

This was one of the many controlled experiences I had in school that conditioned me for my lifelong career as a nurse. Never be afraid to ask questions, no matter how long you have been in this field. There's almost always something new you can learn from every patient and situation.

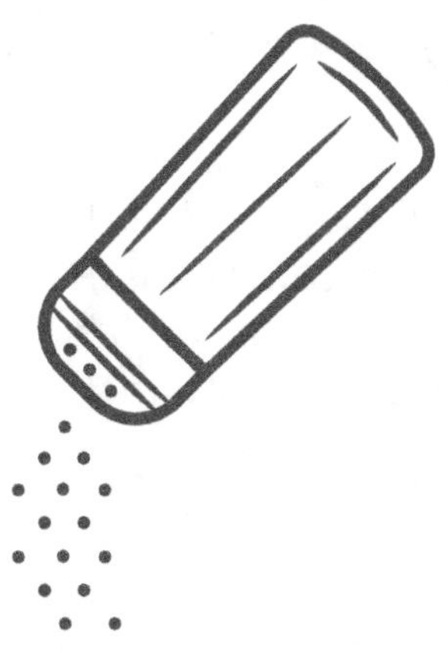

Oh, Poopy

Amanda was a very kind and enjoyable classmate of mine. However, being scatterbrained, you could easily label her as a ditsy blonde. One day, we made our rounds to our assigned patients as student nurses. Upon checking on one of her patients, she realized their bedpan was full and needed to be cleaned. So she removed the pan from its fixed position and approached the hopper room.

Meanwhile, around the corner in an adjoining hallway, one of our hospital's world-renowned medical surgeons was guiding and teaching residents as they made their way down the hallway. As a determined Amanda whipped into the adjoining hall, she was immediately involved in a head-on collision with the medical surgeon himself.

The nasty substance sloshed everywhere, turning their medical whites a saturated brown. Amanda's worst nightmare became a reality as she stood frozen, gazing at the drenched surgeon. He was fuming and glaring at her. As I exited my patient's room, my gaze caught the debacle that had just ensued.

"Oh, God! - How am I covered in this shit?" The surgeon blared. The once lively, bustling group was now hushed and did not dare chuckle or laugh at their inconvenienced instructor. Horridly embarrassed, Amanda could only sheepishly mutter, "I'm sorry." Upon her response, she made a quick getaway for the washroom. The whole situation was a mess.

Though it was a humorous scene, I did feel bad for Amanda. What happened wasn't intentional. Regardless, the medical surgeon filed a report on Amanda, and our instructors made her face her poopy victim and give him a formal apology.

Oh, Poopy (continued)

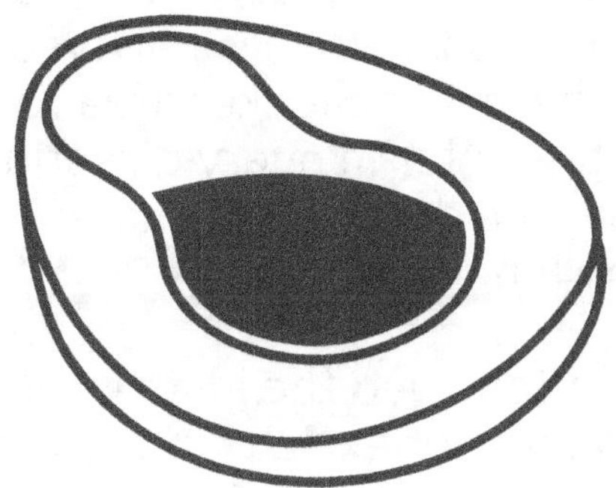

Dr. Frankenstein's Lair

We were told we would have much hands-on training on our first day of anatomy class. When we arrived at the large campus building, there was a locker area to the side and a series of large metal tables in every direction. As we all filled the entryway, the doctor bade us to make our way towards one of the inner rooms.

Once everyone had followed the instructor into a large room, she stood behind one of the many tables and set his foot upon a pedal near the base. Once he applied ample pressure upon the pedal, the sound of mechanisms came into play as the tabletop opened up to showcase its hidden contents. We came to realize all of these "tables" were vats.

To our surprise, a cadaver came into view, and of course, being only seventeen years of age, I thought, 'What the heck is that? What is it doing in there?' Seeing the sea of shocked expressions, the doctor announced, "You'll all be working on cadavers just like this in the future. Any questions?" Immediately, a wave of raised hands came into view. I had questions myself, but I patiently waited to be called upon.

When it was my turn, I asked, "Are these real people? What will we be doing with these cadavers?" The idea of working on bodies didn't initially sit well with me. The understanding doctor smiled, closed the vat, and responded, "Oh, yes. These were real people. All of the deceased were donated for the study of medicine. You will practice concepts on whatever part of the body you are studying in your other medical studies."

There were twelve total vats in that room. All of them contained male cadavers. Our instructor then motioned for us to follow him into a smaller nearby room that contained

Dr. Frankenstein's Lair (continued)

only female cadavers. He mentioned that we'd start working in this room and branch out to some of the other rooms in the building. Like a guide in a haunted house, the doctor motioned us to follow him again.

As we rounded down a hallway, a rather large-looking fish tank could be seen in the distance. However, as we approached the glass container, we all wanted to squirm. It contained a variety of floating bodies. Our guide within Dr. Frankenstein's Lair then explained that these were all unclaimed bodies from the county that had been donated to the school. *They didn't have as many ways to identify bodies back then.*

The various sights in this building took much work to digest. It was odd, gross, and at first quite unnerving, especially only having lived in a small, rural country town until then. I hoped there weren't any more surprises on our first day of anatomy class. After observing the bobbing corpses of the unclaimed, we were dismissed for lunch. But, as you'd expect, I didn't have much appetite afterward.

As we passed the lockers towards our exit, I was walking at the back of the group. Suddenly, there was a loud, echoing BANG! This initiated my fight-or-flight response as it came from behind me. I ran and screamed, "The bodies are alive! The man is coming behind us!" Within moments, we had all run beyond the exit doors to safety.

Once we settled down, several students asked what I meant by my screams. I expressed, "It was the man the doctor had shown us from the first vat." Within moments of my statement, I was embarrassed by my antics. Was it that cadaver, or just my imagination?

Dr. Frankenstein's Lair (continued)

When we cautiously returned from lunch to investigate the event further, it was explained that a repairman had left a small sledgehammer on top of the lockers. Coincidentally, as we passed the lockers, it fell to the ground, causing my mind to blindly assume there was a thunderous footstep behind me.

After everything was reasonably explained, we had a better sense of security. Don't get me wrong, some aspects of this building were still creepy. For example, another room felt like a dark, morbid museum exhibit that ominously displayed a man's torso that had been cut in half so that you could see the placement of tissues, bones, and organs. The campus presented it as a prized achievement mounted upon the wall everyone wanted to see. I didn't know of many people that would have much interest in the specimen. It was educational but gross.

We were taught how to operate the vats ourselves properly. Eventually, we all became familiar with muscles, tendons, tissues, organs, and bones. Various assignments gave us actual hands-on experience.

It took a while to adjust to this different realm. I never truly felt comfortable amongst so many dead bodies. Previous to this, my seventeen-year-old self had never seen a corpse. I just pushed forward by hyper-fixing on the tasks given. The environment felt like something from the movies, except this was real. We had to touch it!

This environment took some time, especially the unmistakable, potent smell of formaldehyde. The chemical caused all of our specimens to be ice cold. Before practicing on naked bodies, we'd learn our preliminary concepts on smaller entities like frogs and pigs.

Dr. Frankenstein's Lair (continued)

Even the smaller corpses occasionally scared me. For example, the first time I took a scalpel to a frog, its legs twitched in a jumping motion. Talk about muscle memory! Another was when I made a small slit down the stomach of a fetal pig. The darn thing peed on me. The splash of the ghastly liquid caused me to shriek, "These things are alive!"

Eventually, we transitioned to cadavers, where we became familiar with the human body and how it functioned and responded to medical procedures. The experience of working on the dead was still odd, but it was fascinating nonetheless. After some time of working on cadavers, they'd eventually turn into a tattered pile of bones. At their expiration, they would be incinerated and soon replaced with the next round of cadavers.

Any day we had anatomy class, I typically didn't eat lunch. We didn't have much time allocated for lunch anyway. Thirty minutes, to be exact. That wasn't enough time to wait in the ever-long cafeteria line to get our food, wolf it down, and run back to class. I also didn't have much of an appetite to eat on these days either, especially after working on the brains of cadavers. I had a new hesitancy about eating scrambled eggs after that. Regardless, I'm happy that Frankenstein's monster never made his presence known.

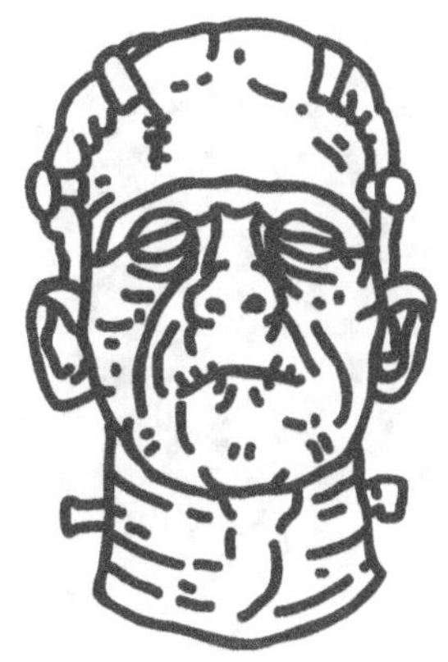

What's Up-Chuck?

One day, I was assigned to the recovery room. One of my patients started to wake. When I checked on him, he lurched forward and spewed vomit all over me with explosive force!

There was no warning and no time to shield myself. I was covered from head to foot. I only dared to breathe through my mouth. I feared inhaling the sour substance on my lips if I breathed through my nose. NO GOOD DEED GOES UNPUNISHED.

I could hear my attire squish and smell the unworldly alkaline stench. My various layers of white were a greenish-brown. All I wanted to do was scream out of disgust. However, I was a student nurse. I had to act accordingly. When the head nurse came over to examine the situation, she directed me to clean the patient, the floor, and myself.

It took some time to get the patient into a new gown and to wipe the sour-smelling chunks from his bed and floor. Unfortunately, I couldn't remove my clothes. I had to remain in uniform. Attempting to make myself look better, I put a loose patient gown over my uniform, but the ghastly stench lingered with me all day. I had to work through it and ignore the foul stares and comments.

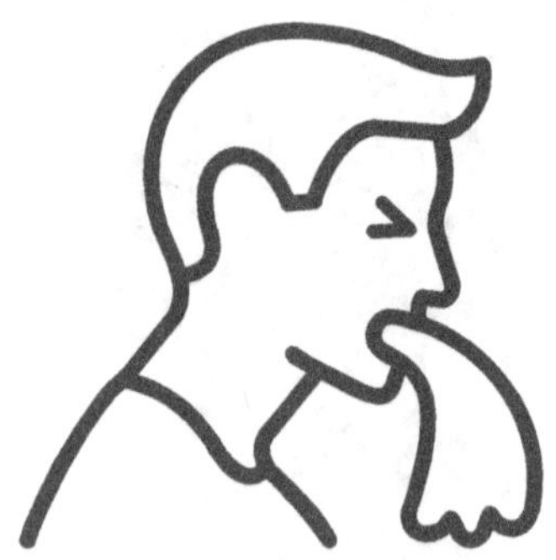

She Was Here...

As students, we were in school for eleven months out of the year. Our one-month break oddly came in August. Once we'd reached our sophomore year in nursing school, we could work in the evening to make some extra money. A lot of us took advantage of that privilege.

One evening, after finishing work, Amanda and Karen headed out of the hospital into Houston's bustling nighttime atmosphere. They were both determined and eager to get home, and they didn't want to wait for the orderly to escort them outside.

Still dressed in uniform, they made strides in crossing the dimly lit four-lane street. The inner city's nightlife sounds had already made their presence known. Karen had taken the lead and passionately divulged her future dreams and aspirations to Amanda, who was following behind. Keeping her eyes forward and still engaged in delivering her vision, Karen suddenly felt a forceful tug at her skirt that threw her off balance. This resulted in her involuntarily falling to the ground, where the air was knocked out of her as a two-fold gust of wind passed by.

Having fallen at the road's edge near the sidewalk, she hastily collected herself and crawled to the safety of the sidewalk. What had just happened? Had someone pushed or pulled her? It was possible. Karen quickly scanned the area for probable clues. There was the typical traffic, but nothing was abnormal, and no one else was around. Wait! Where's Amanda? Where had she gone?

Yet again, Amanda was a fun, ditsy blonde. Had she gone back to the hospital? She was following right behind Karen, wasn't she? Karen stood up, perplexed by the situation. Nothing appeared off kelter, but something didn't feel right.

She Was Here... (continued)

As the remainder of us emerged from the hospital with
security, we all saw the emotional, dumbstruck Karen
across the way hollering to us. "Is Amanda with you? Please,
God, let her be with you!" Immediately, we sensed the fear
and dread that she projected because we hadn't seen
Amanda since the end of work when she and Karen left
together. Security motioned for Karen to stay where she
was as we crossed the street. The guard tried to help calm
her and asked what had happened. Sadly, not many details
or answers came. No one could make sense of the situation.

The following day, Amanda was still nowhere to be found.
She never showed up at work or returned to the dormitory.
We couldn't help but worry about her. It wasn't like her to
disappear.

As we arrived back in the classroom setting, we were met
by instructors and security, which was odd. Security was
never in the conference room. They all carried a somewhat
anxious expression as we all took our seats. As the last
person sat, an eerie silence prevailed before we were all
given the details of what had occurred in the strange fiasco
of the night prior.

In crossing the road, Amanda was struck by a vehicle during
a high-speed chase. No horns were blared. No sirens were
emitted. There was no warning that either car was barreling
towards the crosswalk at a staggering hundred miles an
hour.

The perpetrator had hit Amanda but did not brake or slow
down as the officer remained on his tail. Amanda wasn't run
over, but instead, her poor body was carried for an
additional four blocks, which is why nobody could make
sense of the event in the darkness of night.

She Was Here... (continued)

So, what had momentarily tugged at Karen's nursing uniform before she fell? Was it a terrified Amanda reaching out in a last-ditch attempt to escape the oncoming vehicle? We may never know, but it haunted us. Emotions were at an all-time high throughout the room. We were cautioned about an elongated blood splatter along the roadway. The city was planning on washing it off within the coming days.

Thankfully, the perpetrator did not get away, so justice was inevitably served. Although Amanda wasn't my ride-or-die friend, this event stuck with me through nursing school. I was paranoid any time I crossed the busy street from that moment on. Eventually, the city got someone to clean the street, but they couldn't remove the stain. The horrifying red streak remained a visible omen of the night any time we crossed the road.

We were all invited to be the honor guards at Amanda's funeral. All of us students came in our nursing uniforms. It all felt sad and surreal. As we looked upon Amanda's casket, we knew that this tragedy could've happened to any one of us. Amanda was one of us. She was personable, beautiful, and well-liked among her peers. Now, she was gone. Amanda was buried in her student uniform.

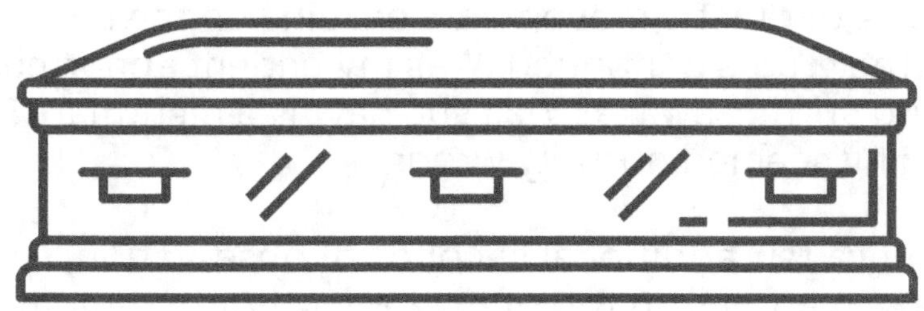

The Despicable Rider

In my senior year of nursing school, I was assigned the acting role of charge nurse on the neuro floor. While starting my rounds, I came to the first patient's room. I had previously read that the patient had come out of surgery that evening, so she shouldn't be awake.

When I approached the patient's door, it was cracked open. There were no lights on in the room. However, I could hear a series of faint grunting coming from the dark abyss. I then wondered if the patient might be making noises while they slept.

As policy directs, I quickly knocked and called, "Hello?" No answer came, but the throaty sound continued. I entered the room so as not to disturb the patient. I only wanted to ensure everything was all right and promptly leave.

When I gave a gentle push, the entryway widened enough to enter. It allowed a few rays of additional light into the room. Now, inside the room, the grunting sounds didn't feel as distant. They were more clear and pronounced. These seemed like odd, peculiar noises for a person who was asleep.

I took a delicate grasp on the privacy curtain and slowly pulled it back to view the patient. To my dismay, I saw a silhouette of drastic movements ensuing on the patient's bed as the grunts continued. Was my patient abnormally large and stirring awake? Was she having a nightmare? Something seemed horridly wrong.

After only a few additional seconds of observation, I realized a man was on top of my patient! At that moment, I didn't care whether the patient was awake. I let out a series of bellowing yelps, saying, "Hey! Stop that right now! Hold on." I could tell my voice had startled this unseen person

The Despicable Rider (continued)

because the vigorous motions and grunting stopped immediately.

I immediately turned around. I didn't know how to react. I wasn't even sure what I had just witnessed. I stepped outside briefly to collect my thoughts and figure out what to do next. When I returned, I recited the policy to this patient's guest. Passing through the curtain, I could tell the man was no longer in the hospital bed. However, that didn't stop me from letting out a stern reminder that there can only be one person in a bed at a time.

I didn't say a word outside of this reminder. I checked the patient's pulse and realized she hadn't been awake—she was fast asleep. What the heck had he been doing? I felt uneasy and promptly left the room.

I spoke to a mentor and explained the situation to her. She said that I'd done the right thing at that moment. No one should be moved after brain surgery. Too many things could go wrong. Throughout the rest of my shift, I checked on this patient repeatedly. I didn't trust that this man would leave the patient alone.

I'll never forget the awkwardness of this experience. Looking back, I realize I was painfully naive to the audacity of the event. This man sexually took advantage of my unconscious patient. No consent was given. It was full-on rape. He was evil. What's worse is I didn't know who this man was. Was he her husband, father, brother, supposed friend, or stranger? I should've asked questions then, but I learned valuable lessons from my mistakes.

You might be asking, 'How did she not know this man was raping her from the beginning?' This event took place in the 60s. I was still an ignorant, innocent virgin. The topic of sex

The Despicable Rider (continued)

 was uncommon in conversation. All I knew about sex was what my teachers in nursing school had put on the chalkboard. She joked, "When you get married, tell your husband to ride'em high." Such humor was wasted on me then.

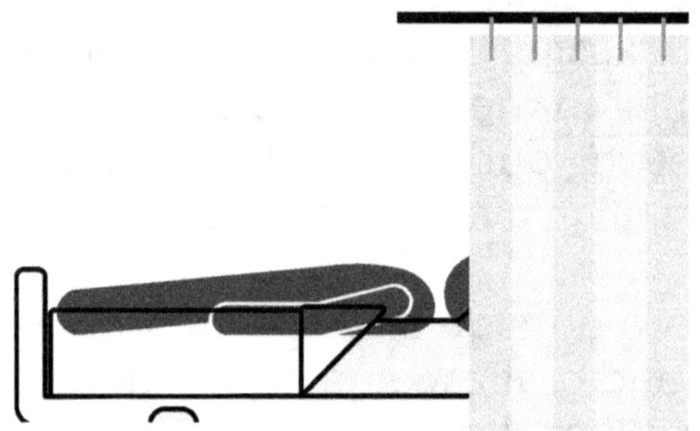

The Old Ways

Many things in the medical field have changed since the beginning of my career. One convenience that has evolved drastically is the distribution of medical oxygen to patients. Today, giving a patient oxygen can be as simple as connecting a tube and nasal cannula to a stationary wall valve and turning it on. You may not have known this, but there is a storage of liquid oxygen accompanied by a vaporizer system that gives ready access to every room within a clinic or hospital.

Providing oxygen hasn't always been this effortless. At the start of my career, when oxygen was needed, I'd go down to storage. Once there, I'd grab a dolly and the large, hefty gas canister. Then I'd run the canister to our floor, offload it, hook up the oxygen, and return the dolly. Without a dolly, moving the oxygen would be nearly impossible. If I had multiple people using oxygen during a shift, I'd make various oxygen runs through my shift to keep up with the demand. After these shifts, my arms and back would be exhausted and sore.

Another item that's evolved is the syringe. The barrel of a syringe used to be glass. After using a syringe, we would reuse them by filing down the needle to rid it of any burrs. Then, we'd sterilize every part of the assembly. Though filing the needle was protocol, people neglected this step because it took time to carry out the act. Because of this, an injection could potentially hurt the patient. Imagine a nurse pulling out the needle of your vaccine, and you feel a barb tugging at you from underneath the skin.

To avoid this unwanted outcome, I would grab alcohol and a sterile sponge and gently run it along the length of the needle. If I felt a tug in the sponge's glide, I knew that a burr was present and would change out the needle before

The Old Ways

administering the medication to the patient. This was the old way, but now there's no need for that. Most injections are disposable because they are one-time uses.

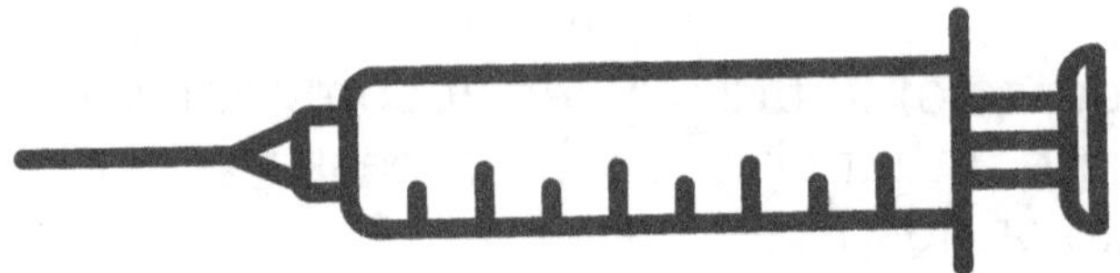

Wheels & Thrills

My first job out of nursing school was at the VA Hospital in Houston. I lived in the women's quarters, which cost me $12 per month. It consisted of a small room and sink. A communal bathroom was across the hall. It was convenient because the VA hospital was on the same property.

It was the first time I'd earned a living. I was paid $3.54 an hour, which was a high wage in Houston then. It was the first time I felt I had actual money to spend.

I was assigned to the psychiatry department. During my shift, I realized that it was time for lunch. Before too long, I found myself exiting the elevator on the first floor and briskly made my way towards the exit door.

Suddenly, I could hear a flurry of noise come from behind me. Little did I know that two grown men were racing each other in their wheelchairs. With both wheelchairs side by side, they were taking up the whole hallway. In hearing the hollering and motion ensuing behind me, I looked over my shoulder and gazed like a deer in the headlights as these two large children were speeding my way. Not knowing what to do, I plastered myself to the side wall to get out of their way.

Then, one of the wheelchair racers came to a screeching halt before me and asked, "Were you scared?" In return, I emphatically stated, "Yea! I didn't want to get trampled." Then he chuckled, grinned, and said, "You would've been all right. As you can see, I can stop on a dime." Feeling somewhat embarrassed, I sheepishly replied, "Yes. Well, I can see that now." I then released my grip on the wall and relaxed.

Something was interesting about this man. His eyes carried a sense of adventure, and his voice was warm and gentle.

23

Wheels &Thrills (continued)

This interaction spurred a lengthy conversation, during which he and his racer companion accompanied me to the cantina for lunch. We enjoyed each other's company and indulged in burgers that cost us ten cents a piece. Can you believe that? While eating, I mentioned that I ate there every day. In the days that followed, Jess, the racer, met me for lunch for some time.

In our various lunch outings, I learned that Jess' upbringing wasn't great. His father hung himself in jail, and his mother was a prostitute. Due to the absence of upright parental figures, his aunt and uncle stepped in to raise him. They had no children but tried to raise him as best as they knew how.

They ran a grocery store in Beaumont, Texas. They sometimes had their hands full with their business and newfound parenthood. Jess established himself as the bad-boy type. He was a jokester and troublemaker. He eventually wound up in a boy's haven.

When he was seventeen, he wanted to join the military but legally couldn't because he wasn't eighteen yet. In wanting to seize the opportunity to help her nephew straighten out his life, his aunt and uncle forged his birthday on his enlistment papers. Before too long, he found himself in the Navy, where he eventually would get hurt while in active service.

After being discharged as a patient, I received a call from a familiar, gentle voice that explained that he and his friend were now living in an apartment. He then invited me to a party that they were hosting.

The party was lovely. The food and the music were great, but the various personalities were even better. Everything was all fun and games until both wheeled crusaders rolled off into the pool! I instantly switched into nurse mode and made strides to rescue them, but their friends jumped in and beat me to the punch.

When both emerged, they only exhibited laughter. Not an ounce of worry was expressed or conveyed. Those two were wild! Their drinking probably only kindled their riotousness. They were the life of the party. Both were hilarious and downright reckless.

In case you were wondering, I wound up marrying Jess. He was a good-looking blonde—a paraplegic who was paralyzed from the torso down. Jess had invited me to another party. While we were there, we mostly talked and laughed together. To my surprise, he pulled out a ring. With a sweet, vulnerable expression, he asked me to marry him. I was elated. There was no hesitation when I exclaimed, "Absolutely, yes!"

He had broken his spine while stationed in Korea due to a motorcycle accident. He was en route to see a potential love interest when his bike slid on a puddle of oil. His unconscious body was found wrapped backward around a nearby tree. After recovering, he would strap his legs to his wheelchair because they tended to jerk and spaz.

I have found that a few nurses married disabled persons because they enjoy caring for them. Honestly, I married him because I just enjoyed being with him.

Though bound to his wheelchair, there was nothing he couldn't do. He just had to do things differently, which made him very inventive and independent. For example, he would maneuver his wheelchair so he could dance fluidly with me. He also made his external catheter.

Wheels & Thrills (continued)

There were not many solutions for disabled persons at that time, especially those who were disabled. When attending a university in Houston, he'd navigate the freight elevators to get to and from classes. For escalators, he tipped his wheelchair back and rode it up or down.

We did all sorts of things together. For example, he'd sit outside and enjoy the view of my heavy self attempting to catch butterflies with a net. He had an interest and passion for insects and would collect them. He would proudly showcase nature's beauty. I enjoyed it, but I was sure he found my struggles entertaining as I chased down each unique butterfly.

Before meeting, the idea that Jess would ever get married had never crossed his mind. Unlike normal males, a person with paraplegia can often have urinary tract infections. Due to this painful inconvenience, he had a vasectomy before meeting me. I'm sure our beautiful, simple adventures seemed euphoric and surreal to him.

Many wondered how sex played into our marriage so that I will be open and honest regarding the topic. Yet again, because he had a vasectomy, we were not able to have children, but that didn't mean we couldn't find pleasure in one another. He was the first person I'd ever had sex with. Due to his physical condition, his erections were random.

We had to be ready for them and act within a moment's notice. Because of his condition, I was always on top. top. Though paralyzed, I wondered if he felt any pleasure or joy in our intimacy, so I asked him. To my surprise, he responded, "Seeing your enjoyment is the only joy I need."

I quickly learned that he wasn't fond of my attempts to

Wheels & Thrills (continued)

 assist him in pushing his wheelchair. He preferred that I walked beside him because I belonged at his side as his wife. I later realized that even though he was paralyzed for some time, he still wasn't very accepting of his situation. I came to know this from his consistent drinking binges.

When I questioned the reasoning for his drinking, he stated that he liked the taste of whiskey. However, I felt that there was more of an underlying reason for the problem. When we first got married, he had stopped drinking. Cold turkey! But a year later, his demons seemed to creep in again.

After a while, either I got too comfortable or was still too young and naive because I'd bought different elegant bottles of whiskey and displayed them on the window sill of our home. They looked so mesmerizing as the sun gleamed and reflected off of their slick surface. Looking back, it was a stupid idea to bring alcohol home even though he had triumphed over his demons.

He would carefully open a bottle, drink some of its contents, and then add water so it'd appear full. I'm not sure how long this happened, but he fooled me for a while. That is until I noticed the bottles didn't look as dark as before. It seemed rather odd that the contents would discolor that quickly. After all, this wasn't the cheap stuff.

I decided to examine them more closely. They appeared untampered with. I gave them a quick whiff, and they seemed fine, so I set my initial wondering to the side. Not long after, those bottles began to appear much lighter. Then, I figured it out and questioned him on the matter. He fessed up to his wrongdoings, but that didn't stop me from pouring every ounce of liquor we had down the sink. That substance was no longer allowed within the home, even if it did come in a pretty bottle.

I didn't fault my dear husband for drinking. I had no problem with him having the occasional drink. It was the

Wheels & Thrills (continued)

knack that he had to start binge drinking that bothered me. Especially when someone was not there to hold him accountable; his actions had stopped at that moment. However, he had opened the door to a greater quench of thirst that would soon make its presence known.

This occurred when I transitioned to working evenings at the hospital. When I arrived home from my shift, he wasn't there. Unfortunately, these events happened long before cell phones came into play. Otherwise, I would've called him, but that was not the case. That wasn't an option. All we had were landlines.

His disappearance made me anxious and scared me to death because I was clueless as to where he was or why he left. It wasn't until I received a phone call from a bar telling me that my husband was unconscious and that I needed to get him. I then obtained the address to the business and tiredly made my way over to the establishment. I didn't quite know how to feel. I thought he was finished with heavy drinking. All I could feel was disappointment, embarrassment, and sadness.

Upon arriving, I woke my husband, helped him get situated in his wheelchair, and took him back home. I was upset with him for putting himself and me into this unhealthy and unsafe situation. After speaking with him, he divulged that he was ashamed of his actions. However, his words and feelings didn't stop him from succumbing to the same temptation again.

Sadly, this happened on numerous occasions following the initial event. He'd give in, call a cab, and drink up till he blacked out. It came to a point where this consistent behavior didn't sit well with me, and we had quite a few serious talks about the matter. Thankfully, the habit became less consistent and eventually stopped. I finally got to where I could go to work and not worry about him or what he might be doing. We got back to a tranquil phase in our relationship.

Shortly after, we went to Mexico for our first anniversary. We saw amazing sights in Mexico City and Monterrey, but the most fun we had was at the bullfights. Though these fights were in stadiums that weren't wheelchair accessible, the staff was still accommodating. We ended up getting the best seats in the house! They took us underneath the stadium, where the matadors watched in wait before entering the arena.

No rowdy spectators were around us. We had an eye-level view of the brave matadors and their opponents. It was fun and magical. Put simply, it was a good time. The actions of the fight played out like the visual spectacle of a movie.

My husband strived to live as normal of a life as he could and was always striving to become more independent. Anytime he deemed that help was unnecessary, he let me know. He reasoned that I was his wife, not his nurse.

Even though we were living life to the fullest, I occasionally saw that his condition and appearance still bothered him. Anytime we went out, I dressed him in dapper clothes. In these moments, he looked and felt confident. But, once in public, we would catch people whispering, "Aww. What a cute couple. Isn't that a shame?"

Other people's pity always seemed to chap his hide. Many people felt sorry for us, even though there was nothing to be sad about. I loved him the way he was and was proud to be with him. I was happy with him.

Wheels & Thrills (continued)

One night, we attended a Christmas party at work. It was hosted at a prestigious judge's house. It was very fancy. Everybody that was a 'somebody' at the hospital was in attendance. In the middle of our holiday festivities, we caught wind of a terrible wreck that had taken place nearby. Instantly, my nurse's brain switched on. Without much thought, a few others and I left the party and raced to the small-town hospital to assist in any way we could.

No matter how selfless and admirable the act was, I left my husband waiting alone for several hours. Without me there, he felt awkward and out of place—like I had ditched him. Now, don't get me wrong—I shouldn't have left, but if you're in the medical field long enough, your mind goes into autopilot when situations arise.

He was very mad at me. After I returned, it was time to leave, and we fought tenaciously all the way home. He ended up tearing my dress off my shoulder. I had never seen him display that much anger and aggression toward me in our entire marriage. It was unsettling, so I stayed with my father for a week to clear my mind.

When I returned home to make amends with my love, he had packed his belongings. I immediately became an emotional wreck as I begged and pleaded for him to stay. My words were no use. His words still haunt me today as he kept repeating, "You can do better than me. You deserve better." I didn't want 'better'. I wanted him, but he was beyond reasoning.

In very little time, he told me to divorce him after our three-year marriage. I did not want to face the nightmare reality. Neither of us deserved to have it end like this. I tried to draw out the process and hold out on hope, but eventually, I had to give in to his determined wishes to move on.

Wheels & Thrills (continued)

His actions did not precisely follow his words. The divorce papers were initially mailed to Jess, but he did not fill them out. In a second attempt to have him complete the process, the local sheriff delivered a second set of the documents. It quickly became apparent that he was stalling.

After filling out my portion of the documentation, I came by Jess' apartment to drop it off and remind him to complete it. Unfortunately, I found him drunk in his bed. His external catheter was overfilled and had spilled all over the floor. It was a horrid mess, and he forbade me from helping him clean it up. Before I left, he assured me that he would sign the papers.

Due to his inactivity, a court date was set for our divorce to be finalized. On that formidable day, I started my drive to the courthouse only to see Jess driving in the opposite direction. Where was he going? I tried waving and honking my car's horn to get his attention, but it was useless. He was gone.

When I arrived at the courthouse, I was informed that Jess had arrived early and signed the required documents. After a grueling nine-month process, my divorce was finalized. I couldn't help but wonder what would've happened if I had gotten there sooner. The thrills from my man on wheels had ended, but I must confess, even now, I love and miss him uncontrollably.

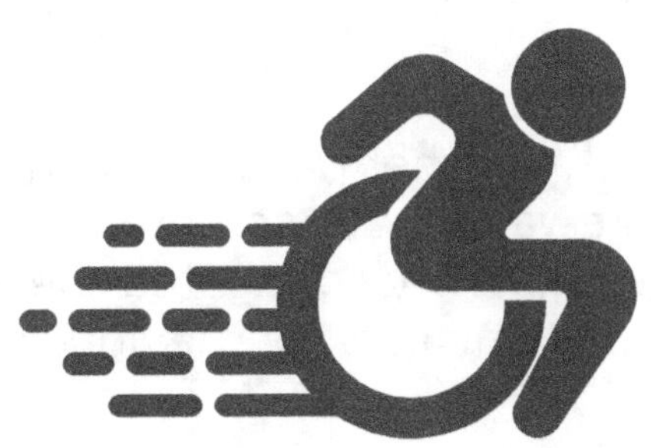

The Cut

Early in my marriage, while working in a small town hospital in the greater Houston area, I had a few interesting experiences, particularly with physicians. *Remember how I said that doctors were treated like hotshot celebrities? Well, that is the case in this tale.*

Jess and I had just moved into the area, and I started working. In the workplace, it didn't take long for me to see who was the highest on the food chain. It was a small town, and the rumors ran rampant. The alpha male was a married doctor who tended to flirt and get around with some of the nursing staff. I would hear the stories from others and see women with bashful expressions as he walked by.

Though I witnessed these daily occurrences, none of his actions seemed geared toward me. Then, one night, while in bed, the phone rang, and I answered it only to hear the voice of the flirtatious doctor on the other end. He asked if I could meet him at his office right away. Stunned that I had received such a call, I looked at my alarm clock to check the time. It was two o'clock in the morning!

Still being as young and naive as I was, I assumed his call was related to work, so I asked, "What is this about?" After my inquiry, there was a brief pause. Only his breathing was heard before he cheerily replied, "You know what this is about." His professional manner disappeared. There was a certain haughtiness in his tone that made me uneasy. Feeling tired and awkward, I said, "I can't go to the office tonight. I need to rest."

From my statement, another pause ensued before he continued, "It can't wait. I have something to show you." As the call progressed, I slowly connected the dots that he was trying to use and play me like the previous other nurses and

The Cut (continued)

I was not going to have any of that. In my stubbornness, I bellowed, "No!" Then, I hung up the phone and retired to my blissful rest.

I was confident that my inattentiveness to his carnal longings would stop these foolish actions from being geared toward me. However, it did the opposite. This doctor unfortunately upped the ante when he pulled me into the doctor's lounge and pressed me against the wall. Against my pleas and with an animalistic nature, he began roughly grasping my breasts. I resisted and did not wish to play along in his fantasies. I wanted nothing to do with him and retreated as quickly as I could.

From then on, I tried to avoid this doctor like the plague. My efforts were useless as I received phone calls every night for weeks. Each night I was getting more frustrated with his antics and I would reaffirm my initial stance from the first call. It got to the point where I finally yelled, "I am never going to come and meet you at your office in the dead ass of night!"

The next day, I began making my rounds, and this doctor quickly came to my side as if he were accompanying me. I felt utterly uncomfortable, and it was difficult not to get agitated. I swiftly rounded the corner and entered one of my patient's rooms to avoid him. I hoped he'd let me be if I remained engaged in work and ignored him. This conscious patient was being prepped for release from a recent surgery, and I needed to check his vitals and take out his sutures.

As I stood on the side of the patient's bed, I caught a glimpse of a brash motion unfolding from the corner of my eye. Instinctively, I shuffled sideways, and a quick, subtle breeze rushed past me. Then I heard a thud resound behind

The Cut (continued)

me as the breeze disappeared. I turned towards the noise and saw a scalpel protruding from the wall.

To my right, I caught the eyes of my wide-eyed, slack-jawed patient. We were both bewildered by what we'd just witnessed. Suddenly, the gentleman fearfully gasped, "What the hell was that about?" In shock, I shrugged my shoulders and shook my head.

I knew then that my tenure at this medical facility would be short-lived. I couldn't go another day like this. My sanity and life were at stake, so I spoke with the Director of Nurses and quit that day. It was the only drama-free option that I could think of. I would likely have been fired anyway for not giving in to the doctor's unethical demands. After leaving the hospital that day, I also felt it necessary to relocate for work once more.

Still, at that time, the culture was that the doctor was always right, no matter what they did. Don't get me wrong; there were plenty of wonderful, great doctors who were true gentlemen. However, there were those who abused their power for pleasure and gain.

This happened when I was only three years into my career. Before this, I was somewhat oblivious to all the foolishness that could transpire in the adult workplace. I had grown up in a rural area and wasn't used to hearing about men picking up women. It was a foreign concept in my sheltered mind.

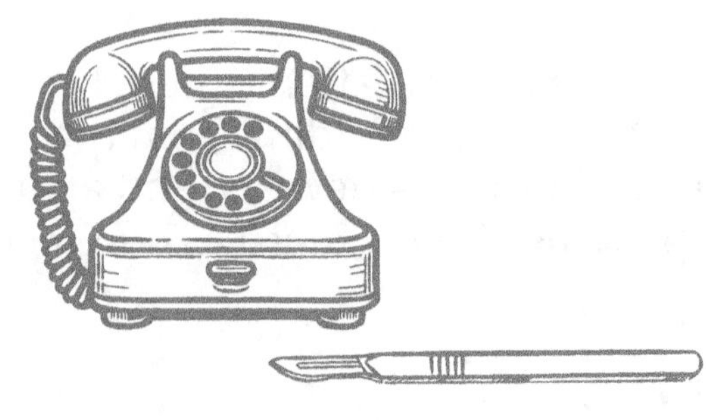

The Old Toss

You may feel that what I'm about to share is unusual and possibly cruel. There was a resident in the nursing home who had an odd heart condition. It was normal for her heart to sporadically start racing, which would make it difficult for her to breathe. Somewhere down the line, a nurse discovered that giving her the old toss allowed her heart to stop its frantic rhythm and correct itself.

So, this became a daily process. Once the resident entered this cardiac state, two nurses would lift her from her wheelchair, one at her head and the other at her feet. Then, in one sweeping motion, they tossed her onto a nearby bed, where the jolting bounce allowed her to regress into a normal state. She'd appear as if nothing had ever happened prior. Though the act was a little entertaining, it proved to work better than any other procedure we'd do.

If you were wondering, these actions were done off-record because, as you'd suspect, any outsider would immediately question the intent of the practice. Am I saying to do things off-record for your patient? No. You should always strive to do things on record. My intention in sharing this is to showcase that we went to great lengths to keep our patients alive. If we could keep our residents around longer in unorthodox ways, so be it.

Now, You See It

At a clinic many years ago, there was a patient who was a small, elderly woman. She was bedridden. As usual, they would take her vitals to ensure she was healthy. After taking her blood pressure, we took her temp using a rectal thermometer.

As a nurse held the patient ready, a fellow nurse was making motions to insert the thermometer into this woman's rectum. However, at the time of insert, the accompanying nurse didn't have a firm enough grip on the thermometer because it was sucked up due to a pending bowel movement. It initially frightened both of them because it simply disappeared. The instrument was there, but then it was suddenly gone. Houdini!

After realizing what had fully transpired, I laughed and gabbed about the awkwardness of the circumstance. Unfortunately, they had to wait for the movement to pass to retrieve the thermometer. To assist the patient in bowel movement, we delicately rolled her back and forth until the movement had cleared.

After securing the fecal matter, they had to rummage about to retrieve the awaited thermometer. A nurse cleaned the thermometer as the other cleaned the patient and her bed. I was thankful that the thermometer came out in one piece and that the woman's feces were somewhat runny.

There was a specific room for cleaning and sanitizing instruments. After a deep wash, they sterilized instruments in an autoclave.

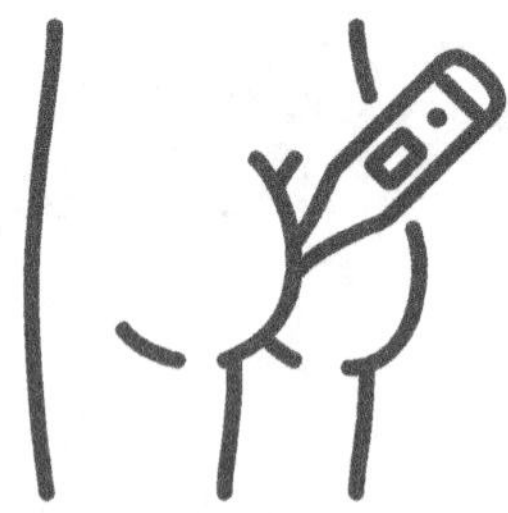

A Frightening Grasp

At the nursing home, an elderly male patient consistently wandered into other residents' beds in the middle of the night. Of course, such actions were not allowed, so the nurses routinely had to escort this seventy-year-old man back to his assigned room.

One night, another nurse made her rounds and noticed this patient's door cracked open. She suspected he had snuck out of his room, so she looked inside to confirm her suspicions. It was then that this nurse had to figure out where this sly man had gone.

Walking down the halls, she looked for any partially open doors. Once she came across one, she'd check on the room's occupants. After investigating several doors, she found him in a woman's bed, which, of course, is an absolute no-no! Thankfully this woman was not currently in her room. He must have seen the vacancy and made himself at home.

When the nurse expressed that he needed to return to his room, she assisted him out of bed. As she wrapped her arm under him, he jolted her backward against the wall with his hand pressed against the nurse's throat. There was a heavy intensity shown in his eyes as his breathing hastened.

Her first thought was to defend herself and hit him. However, she was able to keep her composure and coach him into releasing his grasp. Slowly, he gave in to her commands, released his grasp, and went back to his room.

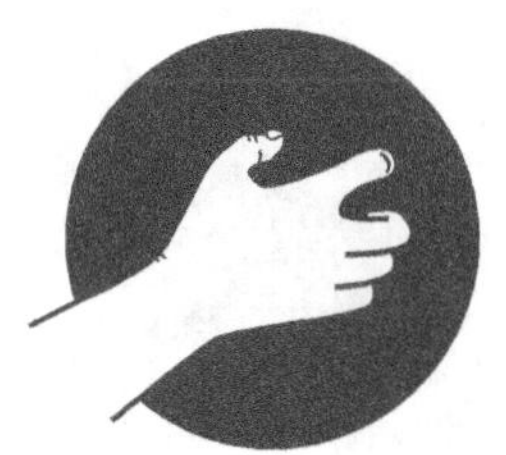

The Two Finger Scoop

Working in a nursing home, you'll find that residents get constipated a lot. We constantly documented whether patients had had bowel movements. If a resident was constipated, we would tend to give them a laxative on the third day. However, if there was no progress by the fifth day, we had to get our hands dirty.

We would have to dig their excrement out with our fingers. Of course, when we carried out this action, we wore gloves, but it didn't make it any less disgusting. After gloving up, we'd turn the patient on their side and pull down their clothes. Once a point of entry was exposed, we'd cautiously put our fingers to work. If the excrement was too large and hard, it needed to be broken up before removing it.

It was a painful ordeal. Our patients would already be uncomfortable from constipation alone, but pushing and pulling two forceful fingers from their anus had them wincing. When doing this, it was an all-hands-on-deck situation to hold their extremities so that the assigned scooper wouldn't be punched or kicked.

We shared a mutualistic relationship with our patients in these events. No one enjoyed conducting and enduring the act. However, if the excrement wasn't removed promptly, the patient's condition could turn grim quickly. As nurses, we did what had to be done. Needless to say, we didn't gain friends any time we had to bring out the two-finger scoop.

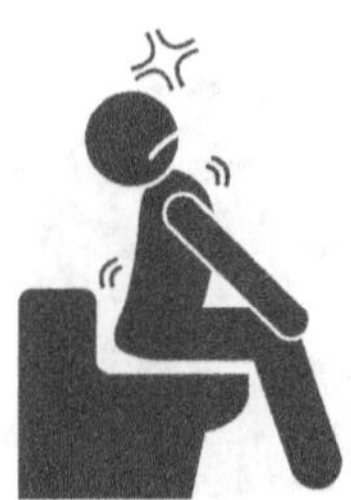

The Selfish, Heartless Truth

I'm changing this a little because this isn't necessarily one experience but a harsh collective reality. I want to state that families don't often care for their elderly. The elderly may occasionally get a visit, but they usually go neglected.

I can't tell you how many times I've called siblings and children on a resident's behalf, begging them to visit their loved ones, and they don't do it. They don't call or come to see them. You have no idea what frustrations and pain our elderly go through daily. They often feel alone, abandoned, and forgotten.

Every once in a while, I will see a person or two who diligently come and interact with their family member, but it's a small drop in the bucket. It's sad and heart-wrenching. Their feelings are constantly hurt. I remember one instance where I caught sight of a woman sitting in a corner weeping. Another nurse came to her side and asked, "Is there anything I can do to help you?" With a trembling jaw and tears streaming down her face, she admitted, "Not unless you can somehow bring my beautiful daughter here."

*I'm going to come out and say it. We have become selfish, heartless people when it comes to looking out for and safeguarding our elderly. People aren't like they used to be when families stuck together through thick and thin. That's all changed. It's a fast world now, and it's easy to get caught up in it. I understand that but know this: **If the tables were reversed, I can guarantee they would make the time to come and visit you.***

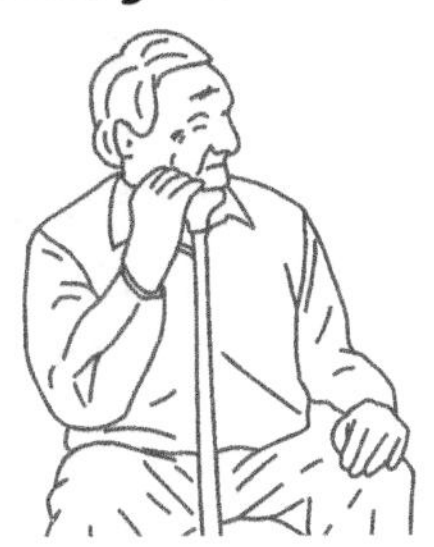

The Insatiable Need

While working for a nursing home, I experienced persons of authority misusing their titles to benefit themselves. Sadly, there have been persons like this in every industry throughout history. Though the work environment and the patients I tended to were great; there was a particular doctor who was very sweet and soft-spoken. I noticed this from the various interactions I'd see him have with other coworkers.

Thankfully, I did not have to interact with him very often. However, there was one instance where I needed to get papers signed for a patient and he wasn't on the floor. He was in his office, so I brought the documents to him. After entering his office, I explained my intrusion and politely asked if he could sign the paperwork. Upon my request, sitting in his armchair, he asked me to bring the papers to him.

As I drew near the side of the desk and handed him the documents, he said, "Well, there's something that you have to do for me." Curious to what he meant, I asked, "What, doctor?" He never responded to my question verbally. Before I knew what was happening, his hands were firmly latched onto my breasts. Feeling them up and down with rough, uncomfortable tugs and pulls.

I did not have the slightest clue as to how I should react to this unconsented action. It was not invited, and it was undoubtedly unwanted! Trying to keep my composure and job, I pled multiple times to sign the papers because I needed to return to the floor. In response, he only grunted, "In a minute-."

After several minutes, I became more firm in my statements, and that is when his insatiable need must have been satisfied because he then proceeded to sign the

The Insatiable Need (continued)

papers and send me on my way. He was like Jekyll and Hyde but had control over the monster, whose appearance was methodically planned. While in public, he maintained his pleasant, inviting demeanor as if nothing significantly wrong had occurred.

I had been violated and abused while in the workplace by a supervisor within the role of a nurse. A role that I hold dearly to as a selfless and sacred calling. I had been defiled, and my views of the grandeur of this establishment had just taken a diminishing blow. Unfortunately, unlike today, there were no resources in the 60s for me to advocate or safeguard myself as a woman and nurse within the workplace. I could not report him without the risk of losing my job. Doctors had full reign. They were perceived as the law and could do no wrong.

Anytime I saw him, I was disgusted and shuddered away from a conversation. Any little interaction I had with him was quick and forced. There were times when I had to get more papers signed, and conveniently enough, he would wait for me in his office to bring the documentation to him. I found myself in these embarrassing, intimidatingly handsy situations every three months for the following two years. The hunger never stopped.

Though it was very unsettling and upsetting, I couldn't help but wonder why he was doing this. This doctor had a family and appeared happily married. It was as if he had given into a carnal state of mind. In these moments, it seemed like he had lost all ethical reasoning. *I often look back at this time and am ashamed I wasn't outspoken about the issue, especially after finding out decades later that this doctor conducted himself in the same manner with other nurses.*

The Insatiable Need (continued)

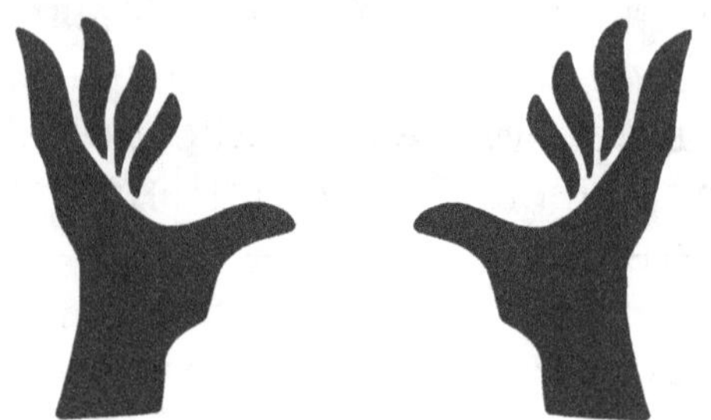

Keep Rockin' Me, Baby

I spent some time in Houston working in the first premature nursery in Texas. Looking back, this was one of my favorite places of employment. While I was working there, a baby smaller than my hand was placed in my care. It was the smallest baby on record, weighing one pound and six ounces.

The baby needed to gain weight while being carefully watched over. The baby was kept in an isolette, also known as an incubator. Isolettes were a relatively new tool, so this was new to me. We kept the baby in an isolette so that we could limit physical contact while closely monitoring the child. If we handled the child, there was the possibility of it losing weight, which would've been life-threatening at that point.

To assist the baby in gaining weight, we delicately gave it one cc of formula every four hours. The 'no contact' mentality made our jobs somewhat difficult but rewarding. Slowly but surely, the child gained weight.

The nursery had many windows, allowing people to see the care given to these little patients. Many people were curious as to why most of these babies lay naked in their isolettes. While they were still in such a small, fragile state, most coverings could be too heavy and impact the quality of the child's breathing, which meant they could only wear cloth diapers.

The downside to not having the baby wear a regular diaper was that pee and poop could get everywhere. So, if the baby got their hands in fecal matter, there would be various brown smears within the isolate. When this happened, on-looking bystanders would tap and bang on the glass to get our attention. They thought we were unaware and didn't know the baby had made a mess.

Keep Rockin' Me, Baby (continued)

Yet again, we had to limit our contact, so we put off cleaning the isolettes until it was necessary. We didn't like waiting, but that's what had to be done. I'm sure some people thought we were neglecting the babies or that we were terrible nurses, but that was not the case. In response to such persons, we would assure them that we knew the baby's situation and thank them.

When we fed them, we would cautiously work around the child to clean any excrement and sanitize the isolette. This meant that some handling occasionally had to occur but had to be kept to a minimum. I'm sure it was tough for these new mothers to gaze through a window and not be able to hold their babies. It was hard for me to hold back from physically loving them. Each of these babies felt like our family because they would be with us for such a lengthy period.

Over time, our record baby gained weight and was successfully discharged. We were always overjoyed when one of our special angels would thrive. Most of them survived. However, a few would not. Thankfully, none passed away on any of the shifts I worked.

A significant contributor to the success we saw with all the premature babies was the use of rock and roll music. Our head nurse showcased this unorthodox practice with us. She explained that when newborn babies are away from their mothers for an extended time, it can be an emotionally damaging experience. To counter this, she would play rock and roll music loudly so that the pulsating, reverberating beat would replicate the mother's heartbeat. It proved to be a great comfort to our little angels.

It was the nineteen-sixties when I worked at this nursery, so we were all into rock and roll. We didn't mind playing that.

Keep Rockin' Me, Baby (continued)

music loud and proud. Amazingly, our head nurse had developed this correlation and the practice independently. It was an exciting and fun time to be alive and a nurse.

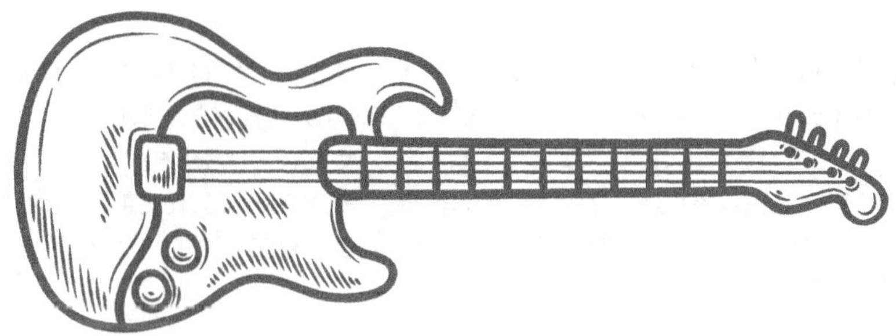

She Knew Voodoo

In Houston, a Cajun woman lived in a condemned building. She was there illegally and wouldn't leave, which delayed the teardown of the house. Regardless of her living situation, she had a large open sore on her leg that we were trying to tend and manage.

One day, while visiting her, I stepped up on the porch where chicken feet hung from the rafters and walked to the door. One apparent thing was that there was salt everywhere. After making my presence known, I asked about the salt. My patient then assured me the salt had been laid to keep the evil spirits away.

I tried not to think much of her response and instead focused on caring for her wound. Unfortunately, after various visits, I quickly came to realize that she would take the bandaged dressing off her leg and leave her wound open and exposed after we'd left. Due to her belief in voodoo and her stubbornness, she'd wind up having maggots in her wound.

Even though I and others insisted that she'd receive more thorough medical care at a facility. She would rebuttal by claiming that she couldn't leave the property. Eventually, because of her lack of care for the wound, our visits became an everyday occurrence.

Hence the phrase, "You can lead a horse to water, but you can't force him to drink." As a nurse, you strive to help people get better, but ultimately, treatment is only as effective as the patient allows. That's something every nurse has to acknowledge and live with.

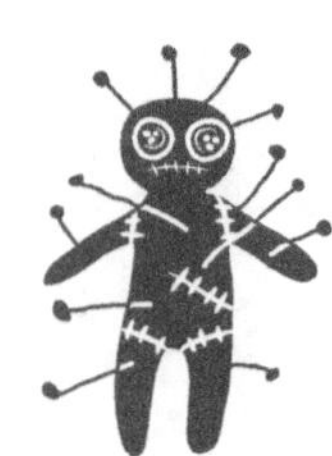

The Flash

In the nineteen-sixties, another nurse was working the night shift at the hospital. When she readied herself to replace the nurses on the previous shift, she suddenly heard someone down the hall exclaim, "Look!" Another person yelled, "Get out of here!"

As the nurse turned to see what the ruckus was about, she saw a buck-naked man sprinting past the hallway intersection. During that time, streakers were very common. They would make a scene and disappear. Maybe they did it all for the thrill.

Everyone in the hospital was shocked, annoyed, or gasping in laughter. It's not every day you see a young man fully exposed, his endowments whipping back and forth with every jolting stride. Within moments, he was gone. The random event caused quite a stir and was a topic of conversation amongst patients and staff throughout the day. Though he was a stranger, we referred to him as The Flash.

The Unforeseen Rebound

A friend introduced me to Carroll, a tall, lean dancing machine. He was a looker who impressed me and brought a breath of fresh air to my life. I even voiced my thoughts about him to my co-workers. I was friends with one of the radiologists. He knew of my exciting romance and jokingly said, "Well, if you're thinking about marrying him, make sure that you marry him away from his mother." His remark caused a funny stir, and I admitted, "Ha. Well, ironically, he lives with his mother." We both gave a friendly chuckle at this fact.

Shortly after, I followed up with the radiologist, exclaiming that Carroll had given me an open invitation to California. I wanted to make a surprise visit. Upon telling him this, he smiled and said, "I guess you better go and see him, then." Then he slid a crisp hundred-dollar bill my way. I was flabbergasted by his kindness and generosity. A hundred dollars was quite a bit of money back then.

Though it was short notice, I asked some friends if they could drop me off at the airport. Once at the airport, I jumped on the next flight to the Golden State. While on this flight, I engaged in conversation with military men who were based out of Malibu. While on the flight, I realized that I hadn't prepped for transportation. Knowing my predicament, these servicemen offered to drive me to my destination. They felt like my intentions and story were worth their time and assistance. I was surprised and grateful for their willingness to help.

It was late in the evening when I stepped out of their vehicle. When I knocked on the door, Carroll's roommate answered while he was sprawled across the floor watching television. As soon as my footloose romantic saw me, he wanted to go out and dance. He then convinced his friends

The Unforeseen Rebound (continued)

to get ready for an impromptu night out.

As soon as everyone was ready, the entire night was an adventurous rush. Everyone seemed excited to take me to the Gaslight Bar. At the bar, we shared a pitcher of beer between the five of us. In casual conversation, part of the group mentioned that we were going to Vegas soon. Confused at the statement, I inquired, "Why are we going to Las Vegas?" Without skipping a beat, they all gleefully exclaimed, "So, you can get married, of course!"

"What? Wait a minute! Is no one going to ask me what I want to do? I didn't even know Carroll that well yet," I responded. There was an awkwardness in the air before his friends chimed, "Well, you will marry him. Won't you?" I didn't know how to respond. Regardless of my feelings, they advised me to mull the idea over while journeying to Sin City.

I was taken to one of those twenty-four-hour courts. As advertised, they made the ceremony as easy as a drive-thru at a fast-food restaurant. Thankfully, we arrived when the clergy was on break eating breakfast. We waited outside the chapel doors, readying ourselves for his return. I was unsure and uneasy about how spontaneous and rushed this all was.

In our wait, I turned to my supposed husband-to-be and stated, "Honestly, I don't know you. I don't think I should be marrying you so soon." He quickly responded, "We made the trip. We're here now. You've got to marry me. It would be a shame to waste a trip." I didn't know what to do or what to think.

The wedding bells chimed in the dawn-lit sky as the chapel doors opened. Cheers filled my ears as his friends.

The Unforeseen Rebound (continued)

applauded the minister's presence. Suddenly, I lost all control of my actions as I was prompted to enter the building and carry out the binding ceremonial ritual. The quick process felt like a raging blur, and before I knew it, I was signing paperwork that made the marriage official.

Afterward, I couldn't believe what had just transpired, and we all had to return home together. While in the car, I sat beside my husband but kept to myself as I tried to wrestle through my feelings. Believe it or not, we barely had enough gas to return home.

When we returned, Carroll's friends dispersed, and we went to a hotel only to crash from exhaustion. That was it. I was married again. I once again had someone who loved me and who loved to dance. The following day, my new husband went to work, and our routine life came into existence.

Within days, I left for Texas to gather my belongings and bring them to my new life in California. After packing my car, I made the long trek back in my new Mercury Comet. Upon my return, Carroll and I got an apartment where we stayed for a while.

A year into our marriage, I received an unsettling call from my mother telling me that Jess had been killed in a car crash. After receiving this news, I had the same recurring dream for a long time. In this dream, I could see the house I had rented with Jess. After entering the home, the view was dim and vacant. There was only a piano and a dismal, slouched version of Jess behind it. Upon closer examination, it was apparent that Jess had eaten one of his arms off due to an unfailing hunger. It wasn't very pleasant!

The Unforeseen Rebound (continued)

Each time I had this nightmare, I would wake up in a crying fit. I suppose I still had regrets about our divorce. Carroll was understanding of how emotional I was about the matter and would help calm me down. My first year of marriage with Carroll was great, and life in California was wonderful.

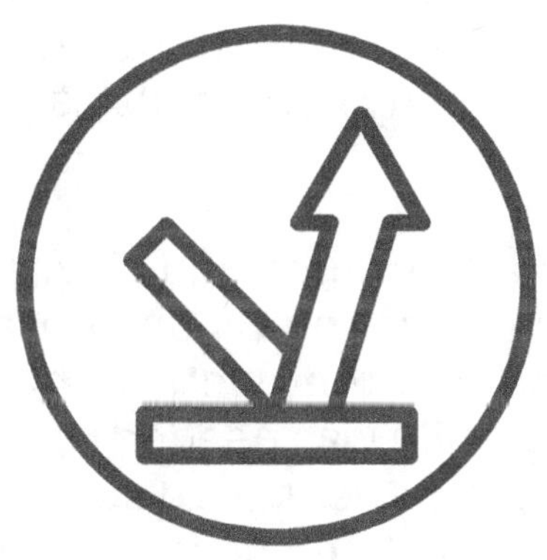

Juicy Fruit

I was pulling into a lonely parking spot at a small hospital in California. I set my vehicle into park, I immediately began my short routine of getting into a mentality that I'd focused on and drawn throughout my career. After a brief minute or two, I exited the car and began taking the brave steps I'd taken numerous times before toward the hospital doors. What would I see or come upon? Nobody knew. I hoped for the best but knew I had to prepare for the worst. There is never an end to how many curveballs can be thrown at you in the medical field.

Upon my arrival, the night nurse quickly reported that a four-year-old boy who was newly diagnosed with diabetes was on the floor and that they were in the process of figuring out which insulin was needed to regulate him. She mentioned that all the patients had slept well through the night and that there had been no problems at all.

After the report, I started my rounds and prioritized the little boy who had previously been mentioned. I knew it was best to check on him first. Entering the boy's room, I thought it was odd that no guardians were present, especially for such a young patient. Regardless, I delightfully chimed, "Good morning."

Silence. No sound or movement came from the boy lying on his back. Without pause, I went over and tried to arouse the boy from his slumber, but he wouldn't wake. Instinctually, I smelled his breath, and it smelled like Juicy Fruit gum. This was a tell-tale sign that he indeed had diabetes. It was especially worrisome that he was not arousing after repeatedly being called to and shaken.

Immediately, I ran to the phone and called the doctor. He

Juicy Fruit (continued)

instructed me to start an IV and that he would get there as quickly as possible. So, I started the IV as instructed. I couldn't help but feel anxious and fearful as I was pregnant and desperately tried to do my part to save another mother's child. Once the doctor arrived, he worked emphatically to bring the little boy back, but after some time, he was forced to admit that the boy was gone. It was too late. He was dead. I was perplexed by the situation.

How had this happened? How long had the boy been this way? This child was supposed to be checked every two hours at a minimum, especially after being recently diagnosed with diabetes. Essentially, this innocent child was dead upon arrival for her shift.

I made the call and coordinated for the parents to come to the hospital to speak with the doctor about 'a problem' that had occurred. I was racked with horror, sadness, and empathy, knowing that this sweet child's parents were receiving the grave news just a few rooms away.

It was by no means how I wanted to start my shift, but I had to press forward. This was my occupation, my calling, and others needed my attention and care. I closed my eyes and held my breath for a moment. At the release, I felt I could compartmentalize my emotions and set them aside.

Would these experiences and emotions come back later to manifest themselves? Yes, but there was work to do and other nurses to assist. People were counting on me. This was all I knew. This was life.

Juicy Fruit (continued)

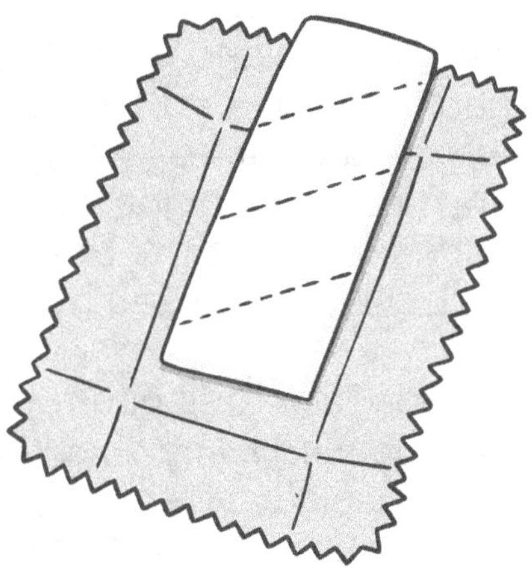

No Rest For The Weary

While in California, I worked up to the delivery of my
second child. The baby decided to come the night of my
scheduled day off. The morning after, I was discharged
from the hospital and was sent home to rest, recuperate,
and tend to my newborn child.

After getting everything situated, I laid my head down, and
a loud, ominous ring came into existence. The phone! Who
could that be? Regardless, I answered it. I didn't want it to
disturb the baby. I asked, "Hello?" A familiar voice on the
other end that sounded agitated and concerned asked,
"Why aren't you at work? Aren't you coming in?"

I was flabbergasted! Did they not know that I just had my
baby and was now on bed rest? I delivered my baby in the
small hospital where I worked. There was nothing
communicated to my supervisors. I started getting agitated
but respectfully explained, "No. I just had my baby last
night." Without pause, my caller claimed, "That shouldn't
stop you. You can still come into work."

I was sure that she was incorrect in saying this and was
saying this out of desperation and stress. Yet again, this
was a small hospital, and we were often short on staff. To
avoid further tension or conflict, I stated I'd call the doctor
and get his advice. She agreed to the proposed action and
ended the call.

I did not feel in any condition to work; I was exhausted. I
only hoped that the doctor would concur and advise me to
rest. I was confident he would, but I grew a little unsure
after receiving this call from my supervisor.

Quickly, I phoned the doctor. I wanted to rip this band-aid
off as soon as I could. When he answered, I told him who I

No Rest for the Weary (continued)

 was and relayed my situation and the conversation that had just taken place. His reaction showcased that he was just as shocked as I was.

His first words were, "Absolutely not! Your organs aren't where they belong. It would be best if you let your body heal. You cannot go to work, especially this soon." He then reassured me that I was not doing anything wrong and that he would personally speak to the head of my department to get this situation sorted out.

I was grateful that this physician was willing to advocate for the betterment of all his patients, including those who work alongside him. In the medical field, too often, it's go-go-go. Sometimes, we forget to treat ourselves and co-workers like human beings. Yes, our mentality is 'the patient comes first, ' but we seldom view ourselves as the patient.

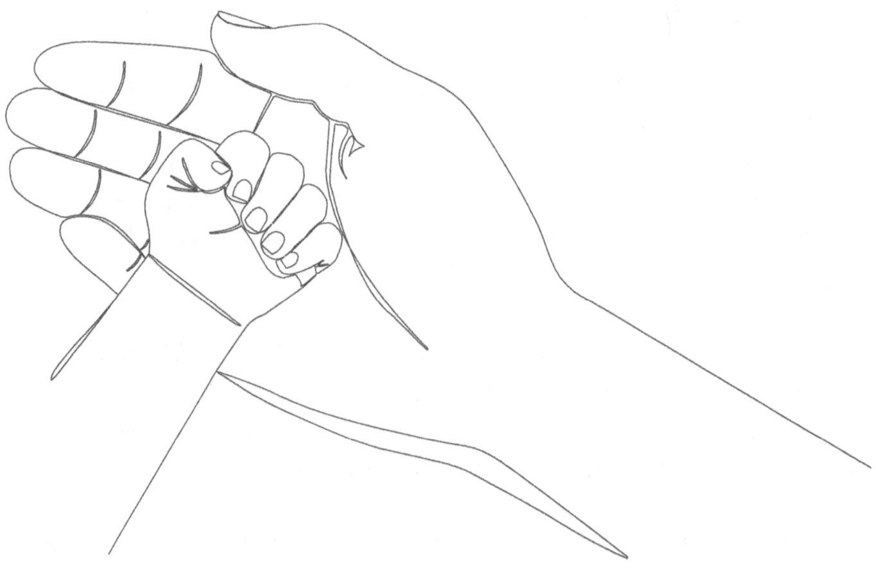

Say It. Don't Spray It

In an emergency room in California, a man who looked to be in his early 50s came in and worriedly stated that he was bleeding from his butt. I accommodated the patient by setting him on the stretcher. In pulling his pants down, I noticed a small, steady stream of blood. I then inquired, " Do you have hemorrhoids?" "No, I don't," the patient responded. "What about intestinal problems?" I questioned further. "Not that I know of," the patient muttered as he winced from the pain.

Perplexed, I then asked, "How did this happen?" The patient sighed, obviously uncomfortable about the situation, and said, "Well, I work at a mechanic shop, and I'm the one that always closes up for the night. I use a highly pressurized water hose to wash off the floor at the end of the day, but I lost it." Confused, I uttered, "You lost it?" What do you mean, 'you lost it.'" The patient quickly responded, "It slipped out of my hands and whipped around, and as I scrambled to find it again, it went right up my butt." I gasped, "What? You've got to be kidding me." The patient winced again as he confirmed, "No, ma'am. I'm not. I don't feel good..."

How had this hose that was whipping around pierced through his clothes? How did the hose get that far up his buttocks? Surely, the water pressure would have pushed the hose back or away before entering this cavity. Something about this seemed fishy, but a more serious matter was at hand.

In gathering my remaining thoughts, I went to get the doctor, worrying that this man might be bleeding internally. Thankfully, I acted when I did because he was and needed to be taken into surgery immediately.

Say It. Don't Spray It (continued)

I never saw or interacted with the patient again during his stay. He was out of her hands. However, I did hear from some of my colleagues that this patient was bleeding internally due to the intestine perforating (exploding) from the water's force coming from the pressurized hose. As a result, the patient had a colostomy.

I didn't know whether this colostomy was temporary or for life, but I was happy knowing that he'd been taken care of in this potentially life-threatening incident. Looking back, I was surprised that the man hadn't lost consciousness from the pain or loss of blood, but I was grateful that I was at the ready. Willing and able to respond to his cries for help.

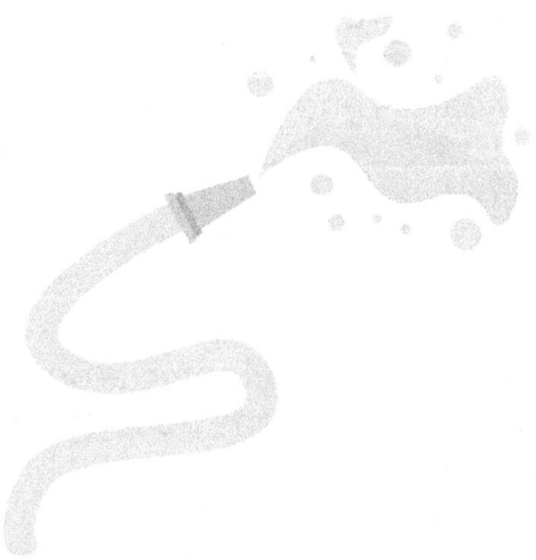

Cumbersome Produce

A man who appeared to be in his fifties came into the Emergency Room with a discomforting frown, saying that he had a "painful problem' and that it needed to get fixed quickly. So, I took him into the evaluating room and asked him what his problem was. He then awkwardly admitted that his rear end was hurting and did not give further explanation.

I found this short statement odd and told him I would need to see his rear to investigate the matter. He agreed and proceeded to lay face down upon the nearby stretcher so that I could pull that portion of his pants down.

After pulling his pants down, I didn't see anything abnormal. So, I decided to separate his buttocks in an attempt to find the patient's problem. To my dismay, there was a portion of a discolored cucumber wedged painfully in his ass. Perplexed by the situation, I asked, "How exactly did that cucumber get there?" The patient anxiously turned beet red before unconfidently responding, "I don't know. I don't know how it happened. It was just there."

At this point, I was desperately holding back giggles and tears. It was a very awkward, random situation. The patient wasn't going to fess up to his actions. I quickly pardoned myself and stated that I needed to fetch the doctor.

As I relayed the details of the situation to the doctor, he exclaimed, "What? Well, I want to talk to him about this." I then led the doctor back to the cucumber patient's evaluation room. As the doctor locked eyes with the sheepish patient, he declared, "That didn't grow there, and it didn't get there by itself!" The patient couldn't do anything but close his eyes and hang his head.

Cumbersome Produce (continued)

"Now, what exactly were you doing?" The doctor pressed for more details. After a subtle gasp, the patient bellowed, "I don't know." The doctor shook his head and chuckled, saying, "Whether you admit it or not, I think you know exactly what you were doing. Things of this shape don't show up in someone's rear by mistake."

With the patient's pants still down, the doctor snapped his gloves on and examined the area of obstruction for a moment. Then, he asked me to keep the cheeks of the patient's buttocks separated. The doctor's focus then turned to the patient, saying, " Now, you might feel some discomfort, sir. I have to maneuver this cucumber to grab hold of it." The patient quickly acknowledged by gasping, "Do what you must. Just hurry."

When I secured the area as instructed, the doctor brought his hand into a cupping shape and placed it over the patient's anus, and began pumping his arm vigorously. With each pump of his arm, the patient would wince and breathe heavily. The doctor's actions created a suction and allowed the cucumber to move slightly downward. Thankfully, there was enough for the doctor to grab onto before it moved again.

"All right. I've got it. Keep him steady." The doctor directed and continued, "Sir, I need you to breathe deeply and slowly. We're not out of the woods quite yet." The doctor then steadied his arms and observed the pace of the patient's breathing. He needed to react upon a healthy exhale and time his actions perfectly.

When the calculated time came, the doctor lunged backward, yanking the lengthy, discolored produce from its dark lodging. It was a success! The cucumber was out and

Cumbersome Produce (continued)

the patient gave an elongated sigh of relief. Immediately, I noticed a few splotches of blood coming from where the cucumber was wedged and motioned my findings to the doctor.

After a quick examination of the irritated area, the doctor told the patient it was best if he remained on the stretcher for a little longer. After the bleeding ceased, the doctor walked with authority around the stretcher so he could speak face-to-face with his deflated patient. The doctor was clearly aggravated at his patient's childish actions.

With some agitation, the doctor stated, "I'm going to put you on an antibiotic, just in case you get an infection. You are free to go home, but you need to take better of yourself. All right?"

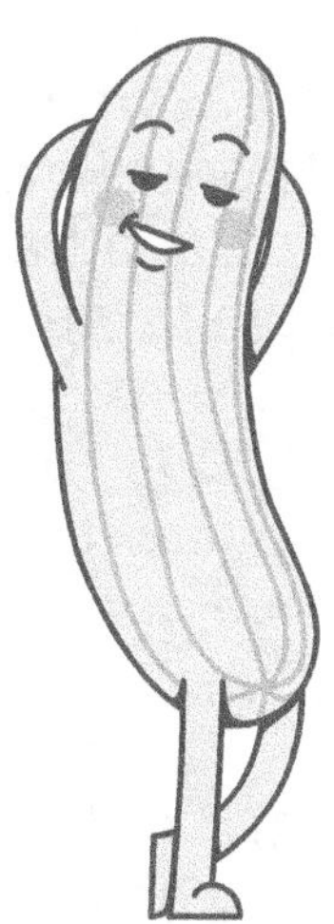

No Class With Glass

A woman in her thirties entered the emergency room in an odd, funny way. I noticed this and immediately asked, "Are you okay?" Nonchalantly, she explained that a Coke bottle in her vagina. Upon hearing the woman's predicament, I quickly ushered her to an examination room. A certain awkwardness filled the room as I confirmed that the patient did indeed have a glass Coke bottle caught in her vagina.

Only the base of the bottle could be seen at the vagina's opening. It was a wonder how the entire bottle had even gotten up there. I couldn't imagine the discomfort and embarrassment she was enduring with this Coke bottle inside of her.

I curiously questioned, "Have you tried taking it out?" The young woman nodded and whispered, "I have. It won't budge." I did not want to risk the bottle cracking or breaking, so I called the doctor for assistance.

As the doctor walked in, the woman's face immediately became flushed in a man's presence. I immediately stated the details on the patient's behalf and asked the doctor, "Why was the patient unable to pull the bottle out?" Without hesitation, the doctor replied, "A suction might be keeping the bottle in place. Due to the bottle's shape and natural shape of the vaginal cavity, once the bottle had penetrated so far into her vagina created a natural seal around the glass surface."

The physics of the problem didn't make sense to me, but I took the doctor's word for it. As the doctor pulled up a seat to examine the obstruction, he looked at me and declared, "Now, you make sure that you stay in here with me." I chuckled and responded, "I will."

No Class With Glass (continued)

The doctor's declaration seemed to lighten the mood in the room. He knew I wasn't going anywhere, and I had no intention of leaving. I was curious to know how the physician was going to get this bottle out.

In his examination, the doctor felt like the elephant in the room needed to be addressed, "How did this bottle get here?" With an inevitable hesitancy in the woman's voice, she explained that she was naked while cleaning her house and had picked the bottle up from the ground and set it on a nearby table. Shortly after, she saw a fallen picture frame on a shelf above her. The woman had to stand on her tippy toes and lean against the table the bottle sat on so she'd reach the frame's general proximity. However, in her stretching reach, she slipped and landed directly on the bottle resulting in the bottle sliding into her vagina.

Her story didn't add up. Regardless, actions needed to be taken for this woman to gain functionality in her nether region, so the doctor advised that I grab a medium-sized chisel, a hammer, and a thick pad of gauze. Once I returned with these instruments, he paused, looked at his patient, and said, "I am going to break the bottom of the bottle."

The wide-eyed woman gasped and shouted, "I don't want you to do that!" The doctor sighed as he leaned back in his stool before responding, "Then what would you like me to do?" The patient immediately showcased an aggravated expression before shouting, "I want you to get the f---ing bottle out!"

"Look. I cannot simply pull the bottle out. It would be painful and could mess up your reproductive system because the bottle is being held in place by an airtight seal along your cervix. To break the seal, I have to release the air

No Class With Glass (continued)

that's in the bottle. The safest way to do that is to break the bottom. There's no other feasible solution," the doctor stated with a sense of authority. It was apparent he was trying to keep a balanced composure.

The woman then continued with a fiery attitude, declaring, "Well, I don't care! I'm not having any kids anyway."

"That's not the problem… I'm telling you that this is the only way—the only solution. You are free to go somewhere else if you want to, but this is the only thing that can be done," the doctor stated, standing firm with his initial statement.

The tension in the room was starting to become intoxicatingly thick. It was apparent that the patient was weighing her options. In observance, I thought the woman was about to get up and leave. I was unsure how the patient would travel much farther with such an awkward obstruction.

Eventually, the woman begrudgingly agreed to the proposed actions because there was no alternative. Upon her admittance and consent, the doctor warned, "I am going to strive to be gentle, but you might feel some discomfort. Please do not move or flail about."

The woman nodded in acknowledgment. The doctor then advised me on how I could assist in the procedure. He instructed me to slide the gauze under the bottle and around its curvature. That way, it would catch any glass particles that might otherwise cause harm to the patient.

After the pad was nestled in place and the woman was widespread, the doctor lightly set the tip of the chisel along

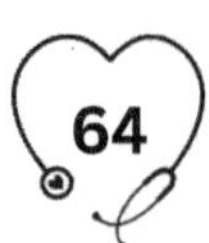

No Class With Glass (continued)

the bottom seam of the bottle and began a series of orchestrated taps with the hammer. The patient and I were nervous about the potential outcome, but we couldn't help but watch the mesmerizing actions unfolding before us.

At the height of the light, feverish taps, the bottom broke off, and the doctor was able gingerly pull the remaining portion of the bottle out of her vagina. As the bottle became exposed, there were sighs of relief all around the room. The gauze pad was delicately removed by the nurse and disposed of. Afterward, there was a quick search for any rebellious, stray glass particles that might've snuck past our sight, but there were none. No harm, no foul!

Even after the procedure, I monitored the patient as she stayed in the hospital overnight. I wanted to make sure that the woman was fine. Although the patient was invited to stay two nights at the hospital, she only stayed for one.

Part of me felt like the woman was rushing to leave the hospital because she didn't want anyone to notice that she had been away and wanted to avoid an embarrassing conversation.

Looking back, I admit I had so much to learn due to my young age as a nurse. That's probably one of the reasons why I can't forget this experience.

After this incident, I found myself opting to drink 7up. I could no longer bring myself to drink Coke. It had nothing to do with the soda. It was just the association of the drink used for selfish pleasure by the patient I tended to long ago.

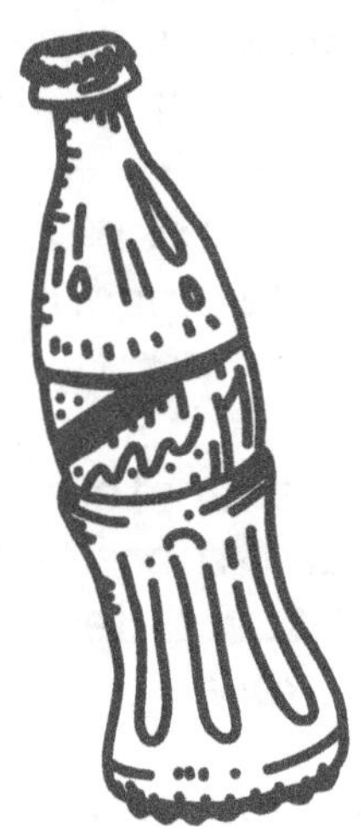

Thinks She's A Somebody

While working in New Orleans, I was assigned to Labor and Delivery. During my shift, I was called over the intercom and directed to make my way to the ER. I thought this was odd, but I was not tending to any patients. Upon arriving in that hospital wing, I could tell they were alarmingly busy.

I then proceeded to assist where the ER staff directed. Not long after, a patient pulled up in what appeared to be a brand-new Cadillac. As the driver's door opened, a woman took her time exiting the car. She couldn't have cared less that she was blocking the drop-off traffic lane. After placing a small, quaint bundle in her arm, she closed the door, left the vehicle parked in front of the ER doors, and entered.

To me, everything about this woman indicated that she was the high-maintenance type. She trotted in with rollers still in her hair, wearing an elegant dress and fuzzy house slippers. Her entrance had already caused a stir amongst the chaos ensuing in the waiting area. When she came to the desk, she said, "The kid's sick." The woman then proceeded to pass the bundle off with an arm outstretched.

I was confused. A child was in that bundle? If so, it had to be incredibly small. I delicately accepted the potentially precious package, opened the covering, and was saddened to see a nearly lifeless child lying hidden in the ruffled folds of the bundle.

It was do or die for this silent, unanimated person, so I and an accompanying nurse dashed to the examining room to further assess the patient. Immediately, she wondered how old her patient was because he didn't have hair on the back of his head and very little on the sides. His skin was dry and wrinkled, showcasing that it was nowhere near hydrated.

Thinks She's A Somebody (continued)

 Matted dirt rested behind his ears and in between the folds of his groin. The circumference of this poor patient's legs couldn't have been larger than a nickel.

Faced with this lowly sight, I needed more details and answers. My temporary companion and I called out to the patient's mother, asking how old the patient was. We were astonished by the response that rang in our ears. In an attitude of being inconvenienced, the woman yelled back, "Ugh. The kid is two!"

We were flabbergasted. This child was a two-year-old? I had seen preemies in better condition than this. It was hard to hold back tears as they now witnessed the result of the painful neglect of a child by someone who had no business being a mother. We had no idea where to start. Time was not on our side, so we called for the doctor.

When the doctor came into the room, he looked over the patient. It didn't take long for him to sour at the child's condition. The doctor's breathing deepened as we reported what we knew. After his assessment, he took a deep breath in before bellowing, "What, what a bitch."

He confirmed our suspicions, saying, "This baby has rarely been fed. It hasn't been picked up or held much at all. This is why most of its hair has rubbed off. It is also apparent that this child has not been bathed or kept in hygienic conditions. Where is this wretched woman, now?"

"She's still outside in the waiting area, sir," my companion responded. There was a brief pause as the doctor rubbed his temples and collected his thoughts. "The nerve of some people. Agh! This bitch is no mother. She's a f---ing monster. She acts like she is 'somebody,' but after I get

Thinks She's A Somebody (continued)

done ripping into her, she'll feel like a nobody."

Determined, he briskly walked towards the exit and turned around to say, "Ladies, this child's condition is bleak and grave, but we have to try something. While I'm speaking to this woman, search for the smallest catheter that you can find. We need to check on the child's kidneys to know how to proceed."

I could hear the doctor belting and yelling at the mother as I feverishly searched for a catheter that was small enough for the poor child. Meanwhile, my companion was watching over the patient. Trying to keep him warm and alive till we could render him service. There was some satisfaction in envisioning this woman's momentary discomfort as the doctor verbally railed into her. Still, it was nothing compared to the lasting disservice and discomfort that she had caused her poor child.

Thankfully, it didn't take long to find a suitable catheter. As we returned to the room, so did the doctor. With a disgusted look on his face, he declared, "As sure as there is a God, there is surely evil in this world. She doesn't care that her child is dying. She only whined that she wouldn't have time for anything if she cared for the child. Pardon my language, but she's a welfare-using piece of shit."

"Those were our thoughts, exactly," I agreed. Turning their attention back to their patient, they noticed his small, limp body hadn't moved. There were no cries of desperation, only limited, shallow breathing. "Let's start the catheter. He might be past the point of no return, but we'll fight to give him a fighting chance," the doctor directed.

With the doctor's guidance, I set the catheter in place. The

Thinks She's A Somebody (continued)

action was easier said than done since the child was the size of a newborn. He was clearly frail as I worked around his dry, shriveling skin. After some patient maneuvering and skill in dexterity, I got it in. Immediately, I breathed a sigh of relief, but we weren't out of the woods yet.

"Anything coming out? His kidneys need to have some function for him to survive," the doctor stated. Due to the lack of movement, I shuddered, "Nothing, yet." After a few moments, I almost got giddy as I saw some movement from the tube. However, it was nothing to be happy about. Optimistically, we hoped to see a faint stream of gold. Instead, we saw five residual drops of urine that had the coloration of mud. Truthfully, I was not confident that it was urine at all. The atmosphere of the room changed at that moment, and the patient gave up his last breath.

His lack of urine proved how dehydrated he indeed was. His life had been hanging by a thread, but now this pure, innocent soul was gone. The raw moment was overwhelming as a flood of mixed feelings emerged.

These emotions ate at me for some time because, at that time, I had two small children of my own. Needless to say, I was anxious to ensure they were constantly fed and hydrated from that time on.

Reading the room, the doctor assured us that this child's death was not on us. It was on the murderer who eagerly sat in the waiting room waiting to see her child out of this life. He cursed her name and vowed to hold her accountable for her cruelty and neglectful murder of the child. He put in an order to the coroner to examine the deceased child so that he could obtain any evidence needed to file charges against the wretch.

Still fuming that this woman had failed to allow this child to thrive, he marched out of the room and let another verbal banter ensue. As predicted, she was not saddened but gleeful that her child was no longer her inconvenience. After that, an evil incarnate returned to her Cadillac for a quick getaway. I learned this horrid woman was later apprehended by law enforcement and eventually received her 'just' desserts.

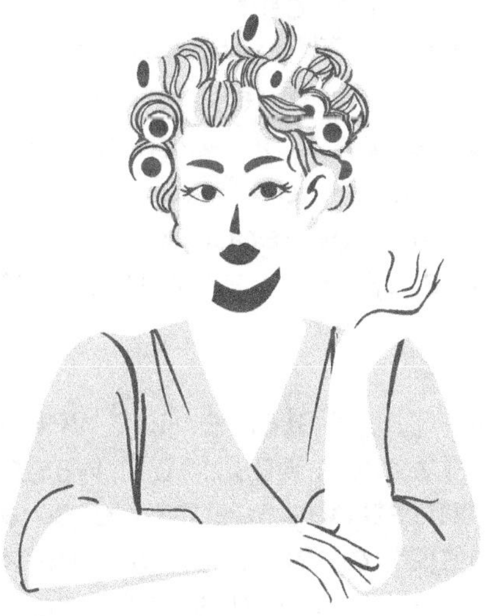

The Red Station Wagon

One dark, frigid night, a man parked his car near the ER and came in exclaiming that his wife was pregnant. Being the on-duty nurse, I immediately sprang into action by grabbing a wheelchair and heading to the vehicle. I didn't see anyone sitting in the front passenger seat of the station wagon, so I assumed the woman must've been in the backseat.

As soon as I opened the rear door, the thick, musty stench of blood and amniotic fluid filled my nostrils. At that moment, I knew the situation had to be far graver than this man had initially stated. The woman was well into labor and was already too far into the delivery process to be moved. Looking back, this was one of the grossest settings I had ever been thrown into. I had no issues with delivering babies. I had years of experience working in Labor and Delivery in New Orleans. However, this setting was different.

Delivery rooms were airy, sterile, and well-ventilated. The back of this station wagon was not. It was muggy, stagnant, and unsterile. All the strong scents were nauseating, and it was impossible to stay clean because the floor and fabric seats were a red, saturated mess. It was all over the place! I thought the husband would've been more descriptive about his wife's situation. One thing was certain, this baby had to be delivered where the mother lay sprawled upon the backseat.

If I'd known the mother's situation beforehand, she would've brought someone to assist me. I was in awe that the man didn't even follow or accompany me to the vehicle where he'd left his pregnant wife. Though I wasn't prepared, for this unforeseen circumstance, I had to switch mental gears and help deliver this unborn child swiftly.

Situating myself on the moist, squishy seats, I assessed the

The Red Station Wagon (continued)

the mother and found that the baby was already crowning. It was clear that the mother was cold as her teeth were chattering uncontrollably. With every contraction, I could tell the mother was reluctant to push as she screamed while straining to hold back.

Immediately, I got stern, saying, "Mom, listen. It's time to get this over with. You can't halt nature's course. You are too far along. This baby is coming out now. So, let's push together."

From that point, the woman pushed willingly while I coached her through the process. As a result, it only took thirty minutes to deliver the baby. Upon the baby's arrival, I could tell the newborn was having difficulty breathing. Normally, I'd reach for a bulb to suction any residual mucus out of the child's airway. However, I wasn't equipped with the tools for this impromptu delivery.

Knowing that time was of the essence, I improvised by delicately taking my forefinger and scooping out as much mucus as I could. It was all that I could do at the moment. The use of my finger luckily proved to be a success. With the baby breathing, it quickly became more lively and animated.

Although the variety of smells was rancid and the setting was unideal, it was a beautiful sight. Once I confirmed the mother and baby were in a good state, I quickly returned to the ER.

I needed an instrument to cut the umbilical cord and needed to grab blankets to wrap mom and baby in so that they could remain warm while moving them inside. Upon entering the door, I was met with wide-eyed stares and glances. I knew how I must've looked and smelled as my

The Red Station Wagon (continued)

scrubs had soaked up bodily fluid.

I was content knowing I'd have to endure the remainder of her shift carrying such an appearance and stench. Maybe people would assume that I was dealing with a rather bad period or that my day had been rather rough. Either way, it didn't matter to me. I wasn't worried about what others might think. It didn't matter what they thought. I was on a mission, and nothing else was going to deter me from tending to my patients.

As I passed through the waiting area, I saw the woman's husband idly sitting there without a look of concern on his face. It was frustrating that he hadn't been of much help through this time, but due to the close confines of the vehicle, he probably wouldn't have been of much help anyway. He was merely waiting there for me to bring her in, unbeknownst to him, his child had already been born.

Before running back out, I grabbed a helping hand to help me safely escort the patients inside. At the station wagon, we were able to safely cut the umbilical cord and envelope the mother and baby in warm blankets. To get them out, I held the newborn while the other nurse assisted mom into the wheelchair. It was of no surprise to me the mother's motions seemed almost frail. She was exhausted and was still trying to warm up from the winter cold.

As we walked through the entryway, it was as if the dad came back to life with a rather shocked expression as he exclaimed, "Oh! You already had the baby?" Instinctively, I responded, "Yeah. It would've been nice to know she was already having contractions." The husband sheepishly shrugged as he muttered, "I had no idea. She was just in the backseat."

The Red Station Wagon (continued)

The hospital I was working at was not effectively equipped to take on deliveries such as this, so as a precaution, we transported the parents and the baby by ambulance to a larger facility. They would be able to help the mother's placenta to pass. As they left, I couldn't help but think, 'We were so lucky there hadn't been any complications. That was a true blessing for us and that little family.'

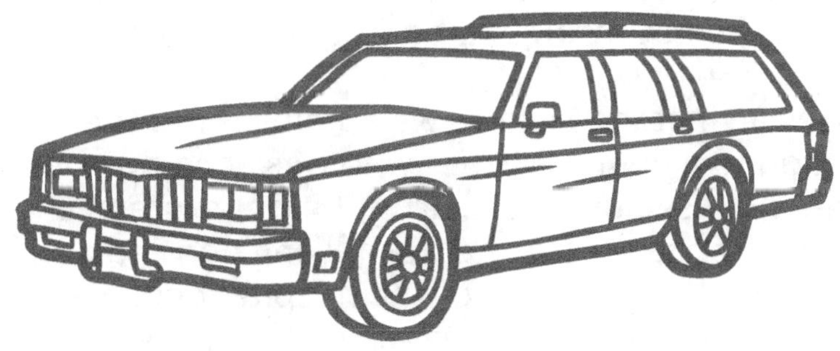

What' cha Know Joe

If you have any experience working in labor and delivery, you'd know that plenty of things are said that simply shouldn't be uttered. Raging hormones, shockwaves of life-threatening pain, and a concourse of mixed emotions can take over and possess any woman who is in labor.

Typically, for pain management, we'd administer a big syringe full of three medications. The combination of these medications sometimes causes women to feel tired and talk more. It didn't necessarily put the mother to sleep, but it allowed her to get through labor more efficiently.

There was an instance where we administered the concoction to a young mother who was accompanied by her husband. As soon as the drugs hit her system, she went into a fiery trance where she was talking non-stop and tried climbing over the guardrail of the hospital bed. It's like she became a different person. Dancing about, she almost lunged forward off the bed, but I was there to catch her.

Immediately, her husband indicated that he would assist in comforting her so she could stay calm. As he drew near, she stretched out her hand and called, "Joe, my love! Come here." Her seductive call caused this gentleman to stop dead in his tracks. The wife continued beckoning, "Baby, I want you. Come be my wild jungle man, Joe."

Wait! Joe? This man's name wasn't Joe! It was Ben! Oh, shit! As I glanced upward towards her husband, I could see his face fidgeting and contorting from the mental flusters he was now enduring. I had to get him out of the room, especially since the patient wouldn't stop bantering about Joe, her mysterious love interest, any time soon.

What' cha Know Joe (continued)

Still holding her, I kindly asked him to leave the room so that I could check to see how dilated Mom was. He thankfully obliged. She still called out for Joe as he made strides towards the door. I felt terrible for this young man. This was supposed to be a memorable bonding experience for them as a couple, but some guy named Joe was dashing it all to pieces.

Once her husband left the room, I could finally calm the mother down and have her rest. That was the wildest reaction I'd ever seen from a patient, and there was no way I was going to administer any more medication to her.

Eventually, through much supervision and coaching, this mother delivered a beautiful, healthy baby girl. After I ensured that mom and baby had settled, I left the room to find her missing husband and inform him of the successful delivery. Thankfully, it didn't take long to find him. He was situated on a bench right down the hall near the nursery.

Anguish and despair personified how he looked kinked forward, his tear-stricken face buried in his trembling hands. He was broken. Like his wife, he was, in a sense, my patient, too. I empathetically patted his shoulder to grab his attention. As I did this, he energetically perked upwards and glared at me before cursing.

I felt sorry for the bloke but was not about to endure an undeserved verbal beating. I assertively cut him off in conversation, exclaiming, "Now, wait just a minute. I had nothing to do with what was said in that room. What I do know is that you now have an adorable little girl. Would you like to come see her?"

What' cha Know Joe (continued)

He wiped his eyes, sniffled, and cleared his throat before responding, "How- How do you know the child is even mine?" Truthfully, I couldn't confidently claim whether he was the biological father or not. I remained unbiased but honest as I said, "I don't know for sure. But as far as I am concerned, you are here. No one else is. This child belongs to you."

I could tell the wheels were turning in his mind as he remained quiet. This was now a moral decision he was making. After a short time gathering his thoughts, he silently walked with me back to the delivery room. His head still hung low. I hoped the sight of the recent miracle would lift his spirits.

As he walked in, he stopped at the foot of the bed and gazed upon his exhausted wife and child. Though he physically showcased little to no emotion, his eyes told a different story. The quiet, reverent scene had brought him into a state of euphoric awe. There was no questioning it; they were his, and he was theirs.

I kept a close eye on them as I continued through the remainder of my shift. Each time I came to check on baby and mom, he seemed to get more caring and nurturing. It was as if he was slowly putting the fiasco to the side, and he'd become the guardian he was meant to be.

In nursing, anything can go drastically wrong at any point in time. Depending on the situation, you can even become the scapegoat and be blamed for everything. You must remember that people are imperfect, and you interact with them while they are in their most uncomfortable, vulnerable state. If they adversely say or do something to you, strive not to take it personally. Of course, safeguard yourself and those around you, but be empathetic and

What' cha Know Joe (continued)

understanding.

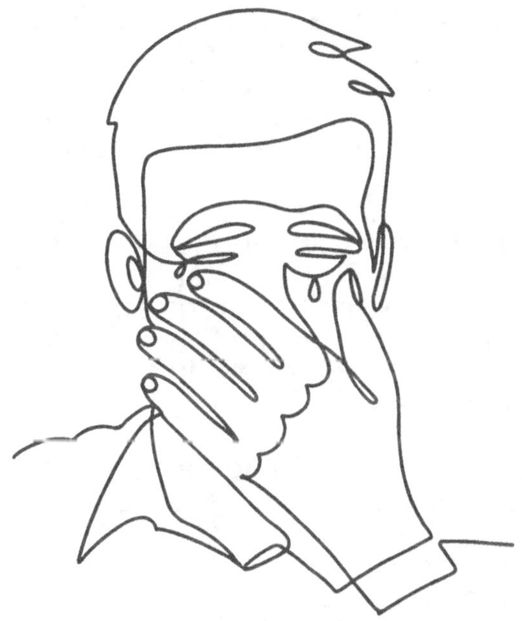

A Mother & Nurse

In Louisiana, Bonnie was one of my supervisor nurses. One day, while at home, she went to use the restroom. After conducting her business, she wiped herself and came across something abnormal. Her unborn child's umbilical cord was hanging out! At that moment, she knew that the cord was probably around her baby's neck. She knew that if her thoughts were true, any movement could potentially increase the hazardous degree of the situation.

Knowing time was of the essence, she had to act fast, and back then, there were no cell phones. Cautiously, through ginger movements, she grabbed her home phone and dialed 9-1-1. After relaying her predicament to emergency personnel, she pushed up against the wall in a handstand position. Doing this would hopefully allow gravity to keep the cord where it was.

It was the best that she could do being alone under these circumstances. This strong mother stood on her head till the ambulance arrived. The very strength and endurance that she exhibited was a fantastic feat! As a safety measure, one of the paramedics used their hand to hold the umbilical cord in place while she was lifted safely onto the stretcher as she was readied for transport. This determined paramedic held the cord in place until this mother/nurse was safely in the hands of hospital personnel.

Once she arrived at a hospital, my supervisor was taken into surgery. Ironically, she was transported to the very hospital where she worked. We didn't initially know that she was admitted to our hospital, but we quickly found out when she was brought into surgery. Due to the nature of this high-risk circumstance, it was safer for the baby to be delivered via C-section rather than vaginally. Enduring through regular labor would put more tension around the child.

I was one of the nurses assisting in her procedure. I was worried for mom and baby's health. We were all especially worried because we knew our patient personally. Bonnie was considered family. It was not an easy C-section either. We had to be very delicate in not tearing the umbilical cord.

A Mother & Nurse (continued)

Once we successfully retrieved the baby, a nurse worked fast to remove the abundance of mucus lodged within the child's airway. All other personnel were tending to complete Mom's surgery.

Thankfully, in the end, all was well. Mother and baby were healthy and well. Before too long, Bonnie was back at work grinding it out like the rest of us while being a new mother. *The roles of mother and nurse are selfless callings. To be both is tough, but by establishing a balanced work culture and good support system, you can fulfill each valiantly.*

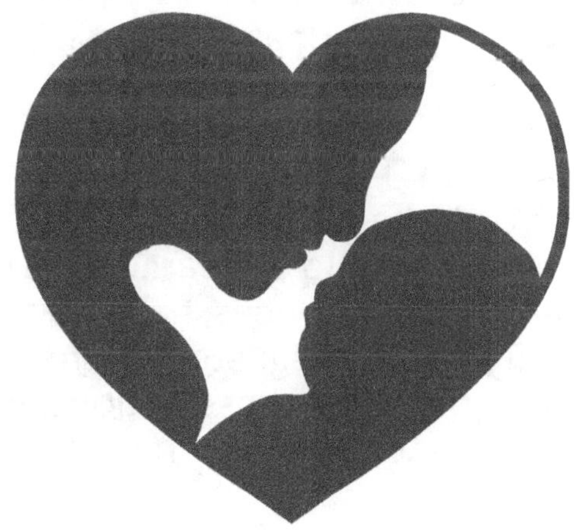

Sorry, Doctor's Orders

Still in New Orleans, I was on the surgical floor and was going through the motions of starting my shift. I saw that one of the patients assigned to me just had a gallbladder removed. As I skimmed over this patient's notes, I was perplexed by the doctor's current order:
"DRAIN SURGICAL AREA. GIVE THE PATIENT TWO OUNCES OF FLUID ORALLY TWICE DAILY. REPEAT FOR THREE DAYS."

I had to read this order several times. I was perplexed by its instructions. Was I reading this correctly? If I was, how was this going to benefit the patient? How would I coax her to drink her bodily fluid? I was unafraid to ask for clarification, so I found the doctor and asked him what he wanted me to do with the patient.

I initially read the order in which he wanted it carried out. He said, "The drainage should appear like dark, green slime. Once you've collected two ounces, have her drink it and repeat it twice daily." I was disgusted by the idea and still didn't know the reasoning for these actions. In my mind, it seemed like such a practice was on the verge of cannibalistic torture.

At the time of this occurrence, nurses were required to wear white dresses that came midway down my calf. With the dress, we also had to wear long, white stockings and a long, thick apron. Our apparel made it challenging to bend and maneuver around patients and medical equipment.

It was also customary to treat superiors, specifically doctors, like kings. Any time they walked into a room we occupied, we were expected to stand while they were in our presence. We were not allowed to question a doctor's orders.

Sorry, Doctor's Orders (continued)

So, in not questioning my superior, I started my rounds. When I came to the gallbladder patient, I tried to mentally ready myself for what I would be doing next. This was my first encounter with this patient, so I didn't know her personality or if she would accept such a vile concoction.

Regardless, I walked and greeted the patient like I usually do. Then, I began asking questions and physically assessing her to ensure she was in good condition. Though it was apparent that her pain medication influenced her, the woman was a kind, older woman.

Then, it was time to carry out the fateful task. Ugh! Just thinking about it made me want to gag, and I didn't have to drink it. I grabbed the container, delicately emptied the drain, and hid my disgusted face as I saw and caught a whiff of the discharge that slowly oozed out. It had a vibrant, slime-green coloration with a texture like puss. I wanted to run at the very stench! It smelled worse than rancid shit or sour vomit.

Once it was empty of the demon excrement, I gathered myself to carry out the almost unspeakable action of getting this poor woman to ingest the substance. Thankfully, she was not all there due to the effects of her medication, so it didn't take much coaxing to get her to swallow. However, as she poured the forbidden juice into her mouth, I had to look away. I couldn't watch it. It was too cringe-worthy.

At her last gulp, she moaned that it didn't taste good, and I believed her. I quickly apologized for the taste. I would not wish the consumption of this upon anyone, but my hands were tied. I had to carry out the doctor's orders. It was awful, and I felt terrible for doing it. I was glad that this wasn't my permanent assigned unit. I couldn't imagine

Sorry, Doctor's Orders (continued)

doing this to somebody's grandma consecutively for three days.

When I left her room, I felt like I had just committed a heinous crime. My appetite was gone, and I couldn't help but think of ways to make ingesting the drainage easier for her. How could I make it taste any better?

I channeled my inner bartender and tried sprucing the slime concoction up with orange juice and a pinch of baking soda. I hoped the baking soda would add a more appealing, fizz-like soda pop. However, my efforts seemed to be in vain. Regardless of what I did, it still smelled rotten, so I continued to give it to her plain.

Truthfully, I'm not sure how she repeatedly drank the substance and kept it down. When it came time to give her a second dose, she expressed her hesitations about drinking the foul liquid again, but she still managed to put forth the willpower to empty the cup. I would have to coax her by saying that it was a necessary medication that she needed to take due to her gallbladder being removed. This elderly woman was a trooper! I felt so bad about putting her through this process multiple times that day. After that day, I was happy to be back in my assigned hospital unit.

As a nurse, one of the things that we were taught to implement was the art of deflection. We weren't allowed to talk to patients or families about their diagnoses. At the time, we couldn't tell them why they were receiving certain medications. We were not to speak about religion. Even though a patient was dying and they wanted confirmation that they were nearing the end of mortality, all we could say was, "No. You'll get better." We, as nurses, knew that

Sorry, Doctor's Orders (continued)

this wasn't necessarily true, but our protocol and policies expressly reserved these topics of conversation for physicians. Nurses were constantly pressed for information, and we could only refer them to the doctor. Thankfully, those policies are different today.

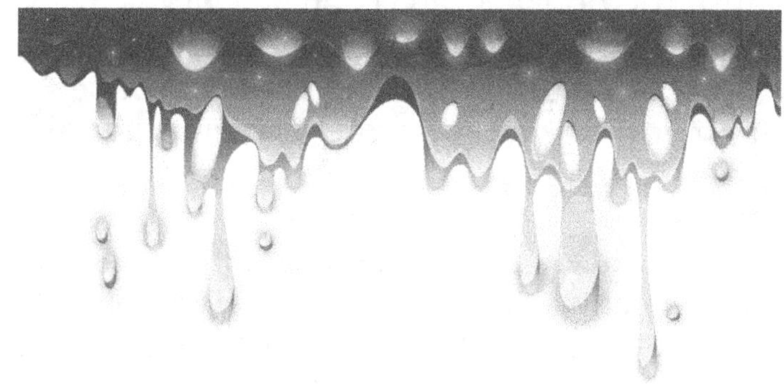

Up To Snuff?

I had a friend whose husband worked offshore. I hadn't seen her in some time, so I decided to stop by and check on her. When I knocked on her door, I was surprised to see her husband, Dick, answer. He greeted me with a smile and invited me inside.

Stepping into the house, I saw a hallway with a living area off the side. A floral couch and loveseat set accompanied a quaint, wood coffee table. "Let me check on Jane. You can have a seat if you'd like," he stated as he motioned towards the couch.

As the guest, I politely sat on the cushion as he quietly walked down a hallway and out of view. The couch was firm but comfortable. Not much time passed before I could hear the sound of footsteps coming closer. Was that Jane? When the footsteps seemed just right outside of view, they stopped. Curious about what was happening, I awkwardly inquired, "Jane? Are you all right?"

It remained quiet till I heard a quick, faint series of metal clinks and ruffling clothing. Something seemed odd. Before I could act, a figure jumped into view. It was Dick! His bare body was exposed, with his pants pulled down to his ankles. He turned to give me a side profile and proudly asked, "Am I up to snuff compared to other sizes, you see?"

I was appalled! I knew what he was implying and trying to show me, but I did not dare look down at his lower extremities. I was not going to entertain his despicable ideas or fantasies. I stayed locked in on his eyes. I wasn't sure what to do, but I knew something had to happen. That loose goose needed to be put back in its cage!

Without much hesitation, I shrieked, "You better pull your trousers up right this instant, mister. Your wife would

Up To Snuff? (continued)

undoubtedly kill if she knew what you were doing." Still, with a prideful expression, he replied, "Settle down. She's tuckered out in the other room."

"I will not have any more of whatever this is. If you don't pull those drawers up this instant, I will tell Jane about this foolery," I firmly declared. I was fuming. This was embarrassing, disgusting, and revolting. As I said these words, a disgruntled smirk spread across his face before replying, "Oh, come on. You're not going to tell her anything." Like a toddler, Dick proceeded to stomp his feet, yank his britches back up, and march out of sight.

He wasn't wrong. I wasn't going to tell Jane. I did not want to strain my relationship with her or cause her any unnecessary stress or anxiety. At that moment, I left and pushed myself to continue my day and not let this incident get the best of me. Though I eventually calmed my nerves and came to see Jane again, it wasn't the same. It became an awkward chore. The fun of having a friend was gone due to the actions of their married partner.

To those who don't know, the public puts nurses in the wrong spot. Due to the nature of our profession, we're never truly comfortable. My grandad told me he'd never let me be a nurse, because 'nice girls' aren't nurses. Regardless of what he said, I remained determined.

My mother also said she didn't want me to become a nurse either. As a result, I carried myself through training and schooling. I had no support. I was my only cheerleader. However, when it came time for my entrance exam, I asked my mother to take me to the testing location. She quickly claimed she wouldn't, so I said I'd walk or hitchhike. Seeing that I wouldn't budge, my mother eventually caved into taking me.

Up To Snuff? (continued)

I suppose people didn't think of nurses as being 'nice girls' because our origins trace back to Florence Nightingale. Though Florence came from a wealthy family, she enlisted prostitutes to help her care for her patients. Talk about tender love and care!

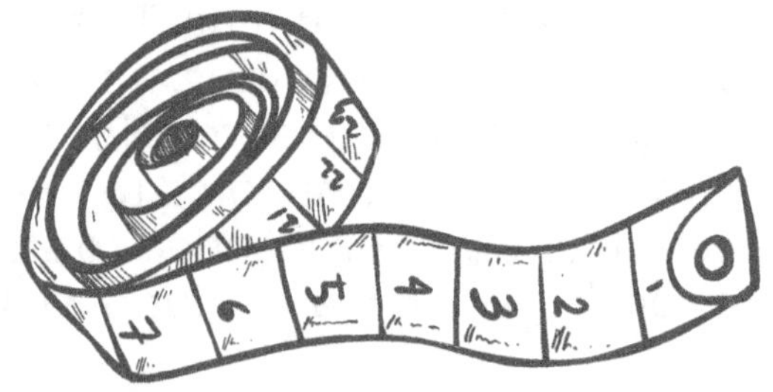

I Didn't See Nothing

On the hospital's surgical floor, a nurse friend of mine was making her rounds, checking in on patients who'd just come out of surgery. She had one patient of Hispanic descent. A few of his family members eagerly waited for him to awaken. Just from the number of people who showed up for the kid, she knew it was going to be a fiesta once the patient woke up.

When my friend came to the patient's door, she could hear quite a commotion coming from within and wondered if he might be awake. The nurse quickly knocked and said, "Hello. "As she proceeded in, she noticed the air felt thick and musty. When casting my eyes around, she saw the multitude of people nestled around the hospital bed talking amongst one another. The nurse couldn't understand what they were saying because they spoke Spanish.

To her surprise, above the group were wisps of thin smoke curling towards the ceiling. "What the blazes is going on here! You can't be passing the peace pipe in here. You'll set off the fire alarm," she shrieked. What was causing the smoke? The patient's family seemed alarmed at her dramatic entrance.

No response came. Only shocked expressions as they parted like the Red Sea. As they did this, the patient and the hospital bed came into view. Off to the side of the bed sat a man maneuvering sizzling strips of fajitas and veggies on his little propane camping grill. It all made sense now!

"No. No! You can't be doing that here," my friend exclaimed as she waved my arms about, motioning toward the cook. Before I could say anything else, a fresh taco was outstretched to me. And do you know what she did after that? The nurse took the damn thing and left! She told me that was the best taco she'd ever had. By time, the nurse

I Didn't See Nothing

had made her rounds to the room again; there was no smoke or trace of cooking. As far as she was concerned, she didn't see nothing.

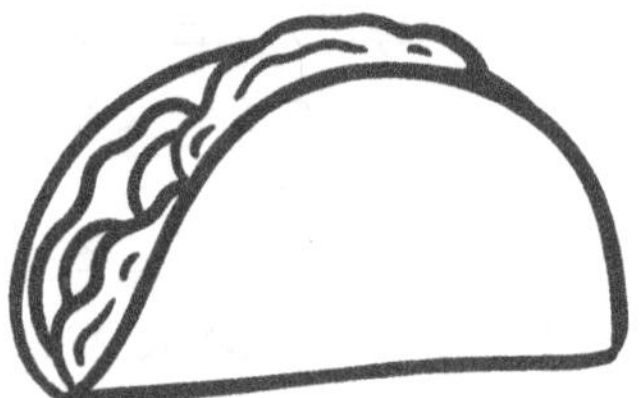

Dead Weight

While in the ER, a nurse friend received a call from one of the doctors relaying that they should expect to receive a body soon. The body needed X-rays for law enforcement purposes. Not many details were shared, so she and three other nurses anticipated the body's arrival. A body coming from a potential accident or crime scene could come in any condition and were typically rough-looking.

When the ambulance arrived with a police escort, they knew their expected assignment had arrived. Quickly and subtly, they rolled the covered patient down to radiation. Before unveiling their patient and fulfilling our service to law enforcement, they gathered all the information and filled out all necessary paperwork.

Once completed and under police supervision, they uncovered the patient in radiology. All four nurses were saddened to see a youthful man who was probably in his twenties. Even in his deceased state, he appeared stout and very handsome. Tidy, gorgeous red hair covered his head and face.

The patient had suffered a life-ending gunshot wound, and law enforcement was trying to determine the trajectory of the bullet's path. Even in unison, they struggled to lift his heavy body from the stretcher and hold him into the proper positions. Thankfully, he was still somewhat limber and hadn't acquired a foul odor. Performing these services with the deceased always felt odd because there wasn't much of a way to honestly 'care' for the patient. All they could do was treat the lifeless shell with respect.

The Scotchguard Infantry

I remember a time in the ER when a young man urgently carried his unconscious friend through the doors. With the limp body in his arms, he exclaimed, "Please! Please help! He's been out of service for a week, and we were having a party…" Tears streamed down his eyes as we came to assist him with the bluish-tinted patient and get them into a room.

The attending young man took a brief moment to gather before proceeding, "He ran around the coffee table a few times and then passed out." After further questioning, the man admitted that they had been spraying Scotch Guard into a brown paper bag at the party and huffing it slowly. I was dumbfounded because of how terrible this action sounded. Sadly, after exhausting our resources, we were not able to resuscitate the patient. This young veteran was deader than a doorknob. What was initially perceived as harmless fun had turned into a horrific disaster.

The doctor had to make a hard phone call to the veteran's family and have them come to the hospital. The veteran's emotional friend stayed there the whole time. Regardless of how irresponsible both parties were, no one could question the person's loyalty to his deceased friend. Once the family had arrived, the doctor took them to a private area and explained the tragedy that had happened to their recently returned son. It was all a sad, stirring example that causes your heart to drop, especially for the elderly parents of the patient. The air was saturated with regret and grief that day.

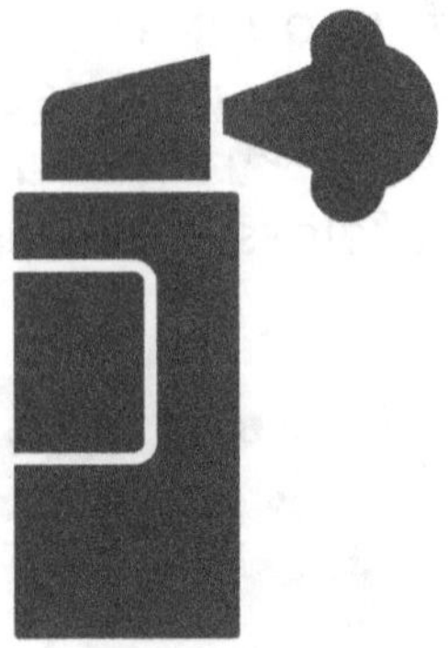

One for You & One for Me.

If you're not careful, this career choice can destroy you. You must have a life outside of work. You must make time for yourself, family, and friends; otherwise, you will lose yourself. Sadly, some nurses succumb to vast entanglements that dwell in our scope of practice. It is a dangerous job that almost seems neverending. Every day, you are always one step away from your breaking point.

One night, a fellow nurse was administering pain meds. She was considered a favorite among the higher-ups. While tending to my assigned patients, I noticed that this other nurse was acting strange. Something about the way she was carrying herself seemed off. It was almost like she was trying to avoid any interaction.

As it turns out, she would routinely carry Demerol, Morphine, Codeine, sterile water, and needles in her pockets. She was the nurse on call if pain management was needed. During her rounds, she would draw out the medicine into an empty vial and replace it with sterile water. After administering the water to the patient, she would then inject the meds into herself in her moments of seclusion.

Please speak out if you ever question your purpose, value, or life. You are not alone. People are more than willing to listen and support you. You are loved.

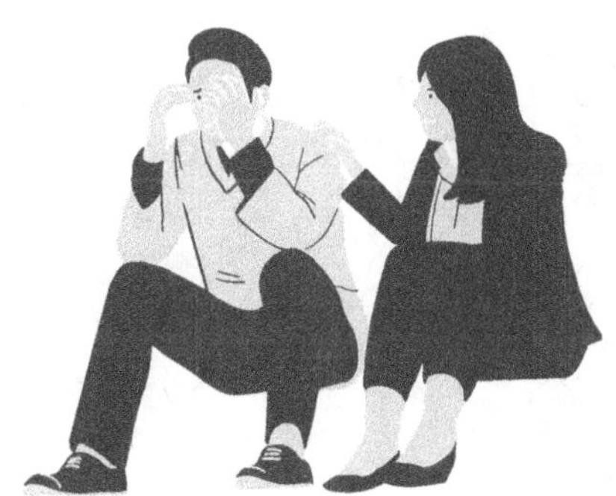

A Little, Wrapped Surprise

One day, I was the head nurse making rounds on the surgical floor. Everything about my shift so far had seemed normal until I entered a patient's room. Inside, there was an odd-looking machine with a bunch of medical paper tape strands coming out of it. It wasn't an EKG machine, and I was perplexed as to what it actually was.

As I progressed into the patient's room, I could follow where the strands led. I was shocked to see that all of the strands eventually encompassed this man's penis. Why was his penis exposed in this manner? What is this a joke? What the hell was this? I didn't know what to think, but I continued acting as if I knew what was happening. Thankfully, this patient was asleep, so he didn't see my alarmed expression.

As I left the room, I called the urologist and inquired about what the patient had been equipped with. He simply explained that a monitor was in place to monitor how many erections this impotent man had while he slept. Ideally, a man is supposed to have at least four while in a state of meaningful sleep.

He assured me that there was nothing to worry about. Everything was in place properly and was being closely monitored. His words calmed my momentary anxiety, but I still felt embarrassed that I wasn't given this knowledge beforehand. I'm not sure why this information wasn't disclosed in the report.

To all you nurses out there, please don't rush through the report. Be thorough. You can save a colleague from headaches or embarrassment, but you could also save a life.

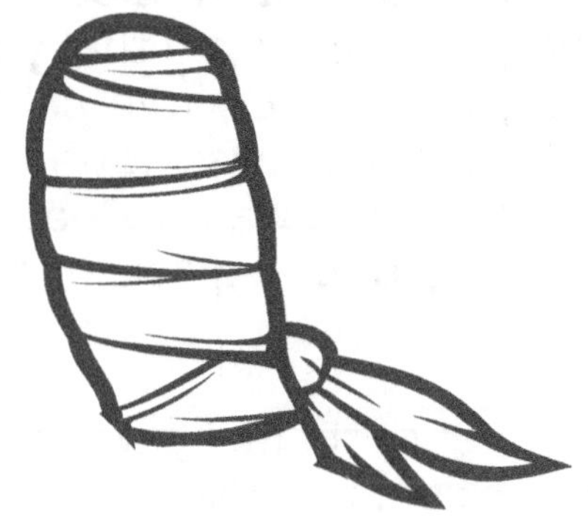

The Truth Bomb

As a home health nurse, I spent my nights doing what people call 'sitting' with a wealthy, elderly woman. In my many talks with her, she expressed that years ago, she fell in love with a young man in the Air Force. As they were preparing for life together, he was notified that he would be deployed soon. They did not want to leave anything undone, so they arranged for a quick marriage before he set out overseas.

Unbeknownst to either of them, he was being sent on a top-secret, classified mission. His objective was to drop "Little Boy," the atomic bomb, on Hiroshima. He was ordered to fly one of the two bomber planes sent in the mission. Both bombers were equipped with an atomic bomb, and one followed the other. There were two bombers because if the first bomber happened to miss their target or went down, the second would act as the insurance policy and hit the target. However, if the first bomber successfully hit the target, the second could turn around and fly away to safety.

After making their proposed drop(s), they were ordered to swiftly fly from the bombing area so they wouldn't be directly hit or affected by the bomb's effects. As it turns out, her husband was the second bomber in this mission. When the first bomber successfully hit its target in Hiroshima, he was advised to head back to base immediately. He had only carried out orders and had little to no prior knowledge of the destructive magnitude and carnage he'd just taken part in.

He was a different man when he came home after being released from his service—no longer a fun, lively, charismatic individual but a dysfunctional alcoholic. The burden had made him sullen. He didn't hardly speak to anyone, and for decades, nobody knew what his service

The Truth Bomb (continued)

had consisted of. It was kept secret to safeguard him and his family from being targeted. However, this took a toll on this married couple and their families. She tried to save her husband and marriage, but it was useless. They eventually separated after years of sticking it out and having several children together.

I was in awe and fascinated that I got to sit with this patient who was connected to such a historical event. The assignment to care for this woman was not wasted on me. No one else had this opportunity, so I am grateful and appreciative that she was willing to share her life story with me.

Unsurprisingly, she explained that people associated with missions such as this were buried in undisclosed places so that no one would dishonor or disturb their graves. And for a long time, even after the wife and kids found out, they did not speak of it.

Though this patient was in her 90s and was recently diagnosed with dementia, I confided in her daughters about their mother's story. They confirmed its truth and validity with their words and countenance. I was flattered that they trusted me with such knowledge. *Even in my later years, their family name will go down with me to the grave.*

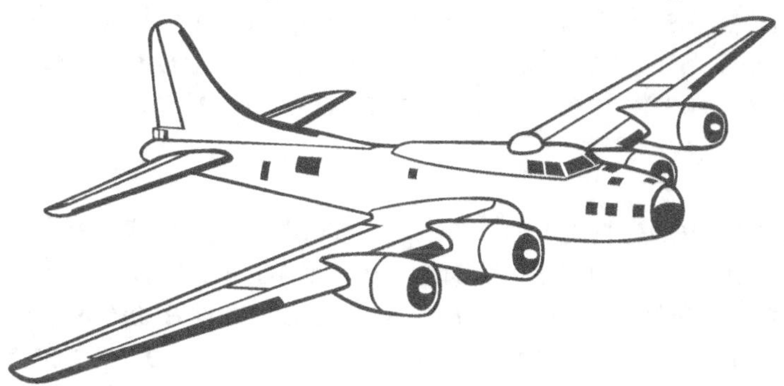

The Devil

One night in the 1980s, a Louisiana fugitive drove across the Texas border, traveling westbound towards Houston. Eventually, in his drive, he found himself in a small, rural town and stopped at a lowly service station. Unfortunately, he had no good intentions as he parked his vehicle. He had carnal urges that he had to itch.

No care or effort was taken to disguise himself, as he was already known and wanted by law enforcement. Plus, he had no intention of sticking around for long. There was only one other vehicle parked along the store, so he was confident that it belonged to a lone employee. Pushing the entry doors open, he remained in calculated observation. Immediately, he noticed an unsuspecting young woman manning the register at the front. She would do the trick.

As he passed through the threshold, he veered off to the right, giving the appearance of perusing the displayed shelves. He was patiently waiting and listening to ensure that he and his next victim were alone. In his meandering, he spotted the establishment's freezer door. After a few cunning moments, the fugitive proceeded to the register to confront his prey.

Now, within her proximity, he played coy, acting the part of an innocent customer as he asked, "Excuse me. Do you have any pussy?" The girl then looked up with a confused expression. She wasn't sure if she had heard the customer correctly, so she inquired, "I'm sorry. What did you say, sir?"

At that moment, the wolf began to shed the sheep's clothing, and a sinister expression spread across his face. He sternly stated, "Oh, I think you heard me. Now, go get in that freezer, bitch." He was serious, and time was of the essence. Before too long, he needed to be on the move

The Devil (continued)

once more.

The young lady didn't know what to do. She couldn't move. What had she just gotten herself into? She was trying to finish her shift and go home. It would be a few hours before she'd be relieved by a co-worker. She was alone.

His subsequent actions were as swift as lightning. He didn't want to waste time. He merely yearned to have his fill. The man lurched forward, grasping a heavy handful of his victim's long, blond hair, and yanked her over the counter before her frightened frame collapsed to the floor in front of him. He could smell it. Control. The power to bend and puppeteer a person into carrying out his will.

This would be all too easy for him. The woman shrieked out in agony and pleaded for her abuser to stop his actions. Sadly, this had the exact opposite effect on her intentions. Unbeknownst to her, she was pouring fuel into the fire. This monster loved to entertain the cat and mouse game. The victim was falling perfectly in line with his vision.

He had no intention of letting her go of her hair. He resumed his tight grip and began stepping towards the freezer door, with the cashier dragged from behind. Adrenaline was pumping through both individuals. For one, it was due to the impending fulfillment of pleasure. For the other, it was the sudden, drastic transition of fearing for her life.

As she heard the ominous unlatching of the freezer door, she began kicking and screaming more loudly. She knew that soon, nobody could see or hear her frantic cries for help. This was her last chance before any remaining hope diminished. She tried to hold onto the metal shelving, but it was useless. Her predator dominated over her through a

The Devil

hefty onslaught of painful pulls and jars. Eventually, she couldn't hold on anymore and was quickly consumed by the dark, frigid abyss.

The frigid air and ice began numbing her extremities. She could see a faint, thin sliver of light protruding from the freezer's doorway. The door wasn't fully closed. Was there a way to escape? Her captor's ever-fervent grasp was still holding her. Before she had time to think, she heard the shuffling of feet around her as her head bobbled from the sporadic movement. As soon as his motions stopped, a thick, frosty breeze was cast across the girl's face. He was hovering over her, taking in the moment and examining her.

The monster then let out a sinister chuckle before drawing close to her ear and whispering, "Alright, young thing. It's time to put you to work." *In an attempt to spare you the grim details of what transpired after that, I will simply say the devil forcibly beat her into submitting to perform oral sex and afterward proceeded to rape her. When satisfied, he fastened his garments, left the beaten girl locked in the freezer, and continued his highway drive. She remained mentally broken and physically exposed until someone eventually heard her cries of distress.*

How do I know this? I was there, sitting in the courtroom while the heinous details of these testimonies were given. Eventually, in this trial, I would take the stand to give my testimony of what I had witnessed, which I will express to you now.

At the time of the crime, I was the supervisor nurse at a small hospital in that area. While making my rounds, I received an urgent call from law enforcement stating they were en route to the hospital. They did not share many

The Devil (continued)

details other than that there was a rape victim who needed to be examined and that they needed me to gather DNA deposits for evidence.

Upon hearing this, I took this assignment upon myself and prepared the room and rape kit for our expected visitor. When they arrived, several officers escorted the patient inside and stood guard outside the door to the examination room. I was the only person allowed to examine her. Everyone was determined not to let anything else happen to her.

At that time, she was still shaking and shivering uncontrollably. As I assisted in removing the various layers of blankets wrapped around her, I quickly realized that she was a gorgeous young woman. I knew she still had to feel vulnerable, so I spoke softly to her and coached and guided her through the evaluation. In the little responses she gave me, she spoke gently, and it was apparent that she was very meek.

There were several moments where she trembled and yelped due to how sore and traumatized she was. But we were able to get through those heavy, delicate moments together. After noting my findings and sealing the DNA evidence, I began carefully cleaning her bruised and tattered body. During this, the darling carried an embarrassed, sheepish expression as if she had done something wrong. I was shocked that she was still frigid to the touch. I did not dare talk about or ask her for any details regarding the event. She'd gone through enough misery, and I was confident law enforcement had already obtained her statement.

Seeing her body and how she carried herself was enough for me. In a way, I already knew what had taken place. That

The Devil

night, I held a piece of her nightmare experience because
night, I carried a piece of her nightmare experience because
I knew the evils that had to transpire to inflict such
irreparable damage. This battered, vulnerable girl stayed in
my prayers, but the look of utter terror remained in my
mind forever.

*Flash forward to when I was summoned to the courtroom.
As I took the stand, I finally caught sight of the convicted
murderer and rapist. Surprisingly, this 40-year-old man's
appearance was well-kept. His style and clothing were
quite dapper when paired with a charming smile. But when
my eyes connected with his, it sent jolting shivers down my
spine. He carried a pair of soulless, ravaging eyes void of
morality. Immediately, I felt like he wanted to kill me. They
were horrible. If I were that girl at the service station that
fateful night, I would have run for the hills when I saw
those eyes.*

*Regardless, I bore solemn testimony of what I'd witnessed.
I remained on the stand for over half an hour as I was
asked to confirm the evidence and my findings that were
presented in the case. At the close of the case, the devil
himself was given the death penalty. The vile creature had
finally been sentenced for his doings.*

*When I finally got home on that hot summer day, I couldn't
help but randomly shutter and shiver. Those hellish eyes
were enough to keep me up at night, and the unrealistic
fear that he'd escape to come and murder me filled my
mind.*

*You might have heard the song, 'The Devil Went Down to
Georgia,' Well, I'm here to tell you that he came down to
Texas, too. As a nurse, there are interactions and
situations that you're thrown into that you'll never be able*

The Devil

to forget. I've seen nurses turn to drugs and drinking in an attempt to douse their cruel memories away or to escape the reality of their craft. Unfortunately, those practices never work.

Though we may not be the direct victims of such travesties, we carry the burden of seeing and knowing the unspeakable. Like most emergency personnel, we suffer heavily from PTSD, and if left untreated, it can wreak havoc on our mental well-being and personal lives. If you are struggling, I strongly advise seeking professional help and guidance. If you do this, you will not be sorry. I speak out of love and experience.

Sometime later in my career, I worked in the prison system and found out that the Devil's sentence had been fulfilled. Receiving this news caused me to sigh in relief as I clapped my hands together. It was finished. The Devil was gone.

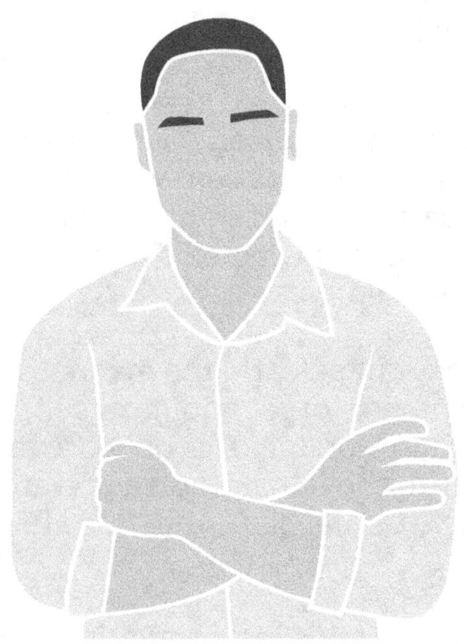

The Weight I Carry

At the beginning of a friend's shift, she received a call that a woman was suffering a stroke and was being brought by ambulance to the hospital. She was present at the patient's arrival and assisted in unloading her off the truck. It quickly became apparent that the patient was already near death and having a hard time breathing. The hospital was already low-staffed, so she alone was trying to stabilize this elderly lady.

This nurse knew that more hands were needed as she repeatedly hit the call button and pleaded for help while holding the woman's head back so that she could breathe more effectively. She screamed for the charge nurse but obtained no response. All staff was utterly stretched thin. In those moments, this nurse knew that this dire situation would not end happily. To no avail, she continued yelling for assistance. Not long after, while on the cusp of death, she felt a subtle stirring vibrate through the patient's body before she was ultimately gone. Had she just experienced the supernatural?

This wasn't the first time she'd seen someone pass, but it was the first time it had caused her to be this unsettled. Though this nurse felt the patient was now in a better place, the incident unearthed a different perspective on life for her. She felt useless, but what else could she have done in that event? It haunted her.

Even after the patient's death, the madness in the ER didn't end. This nurse had to forget about herself, swallow her emotions, and keep working. This only proved to be an adverse catalyst to the initial trauma of watching this woman's death. After her shift, the nurse felt weak and sobbed for hours.

Over time, she re-established confidence in her nursing

The Weight I Carry

skills and purpose. However, events like this only add to the mental weight that all nurses carry. A weight that we will eventually take to our grave.

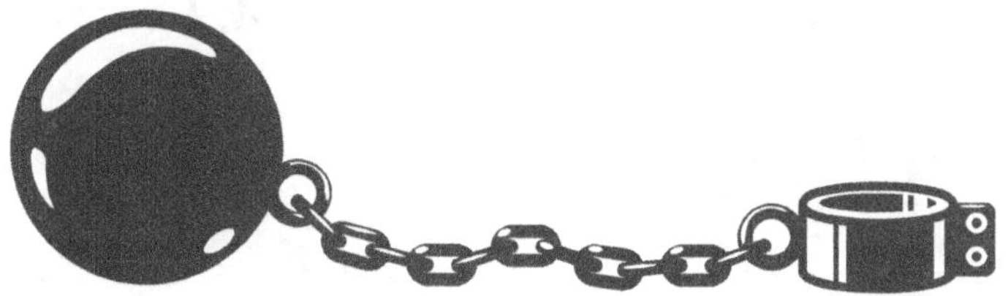

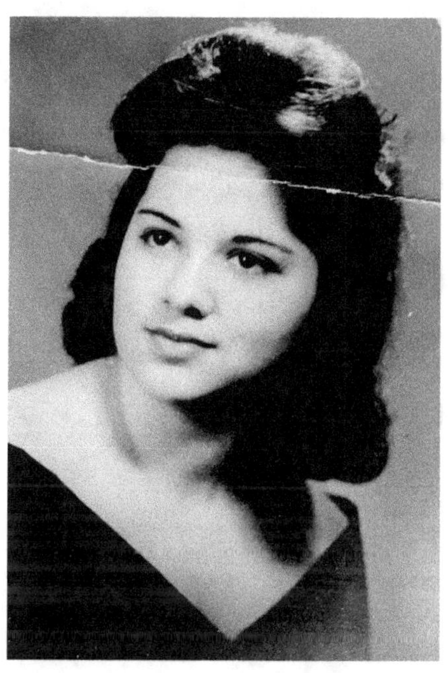

A glamour shot of Lynda.

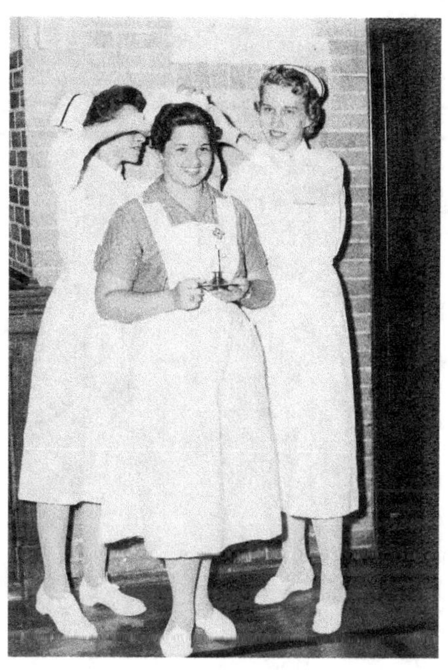

Lynda's pinning ceremony.

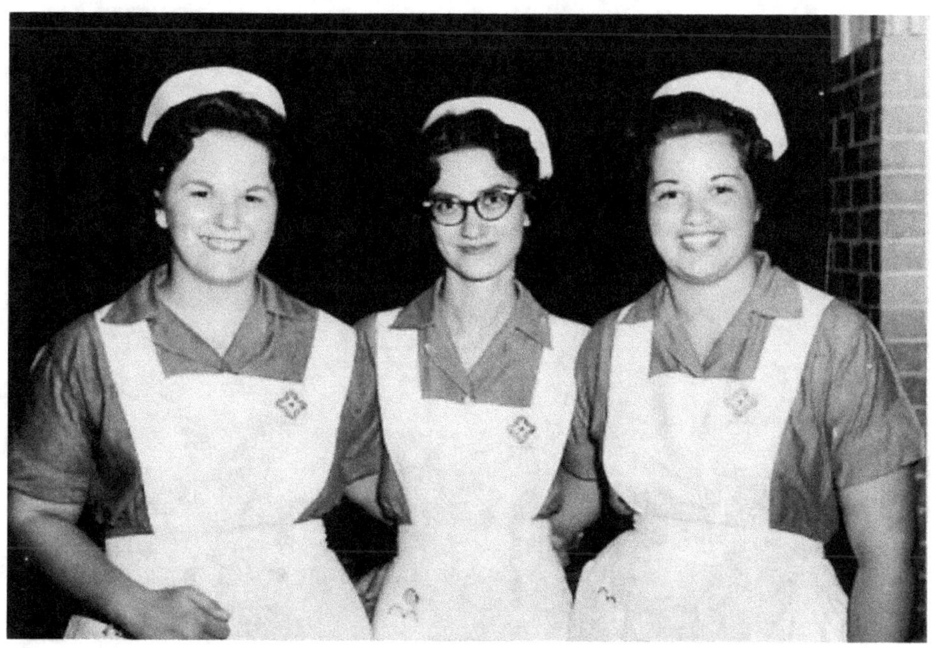

Lynda and a few other graduates after their pinning ceremony.

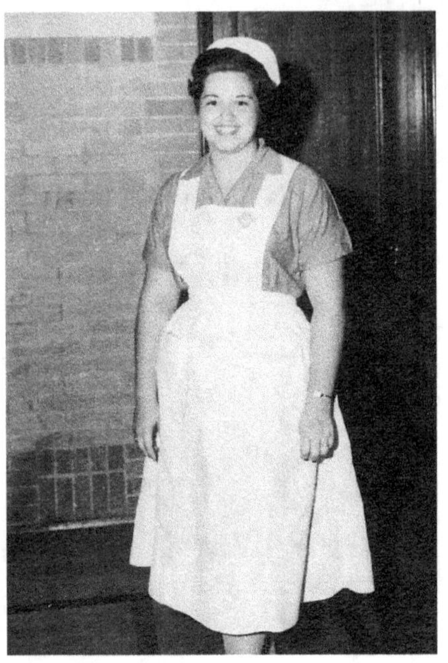

*Lynda posing after
becoming a nurse.*

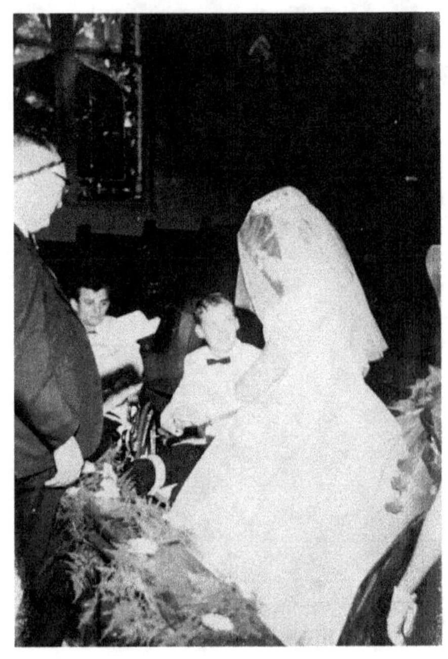

*Lynda and Jess preparing
to give their vows.*

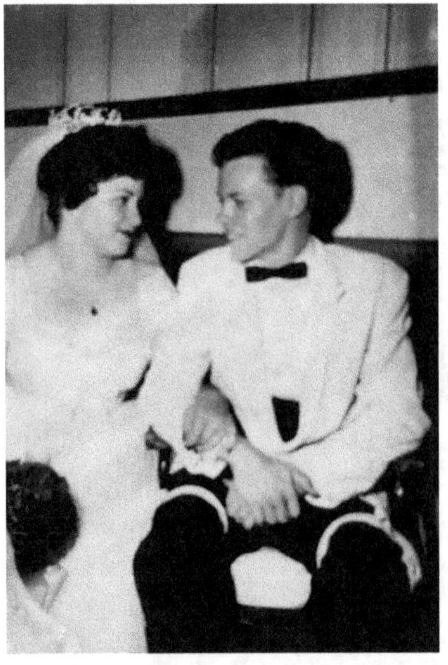

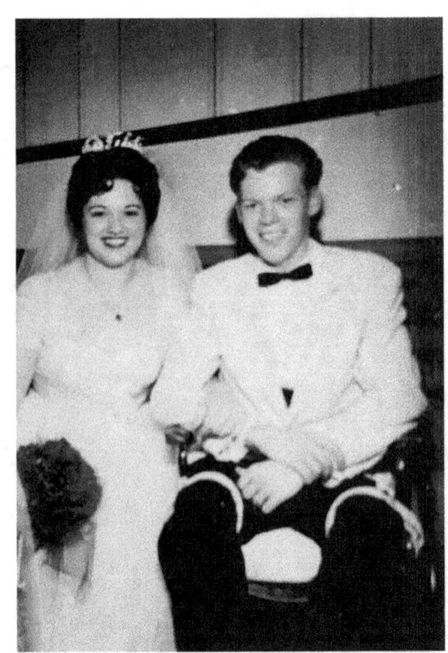

Lynda and Jess happily posing on their wedding day.

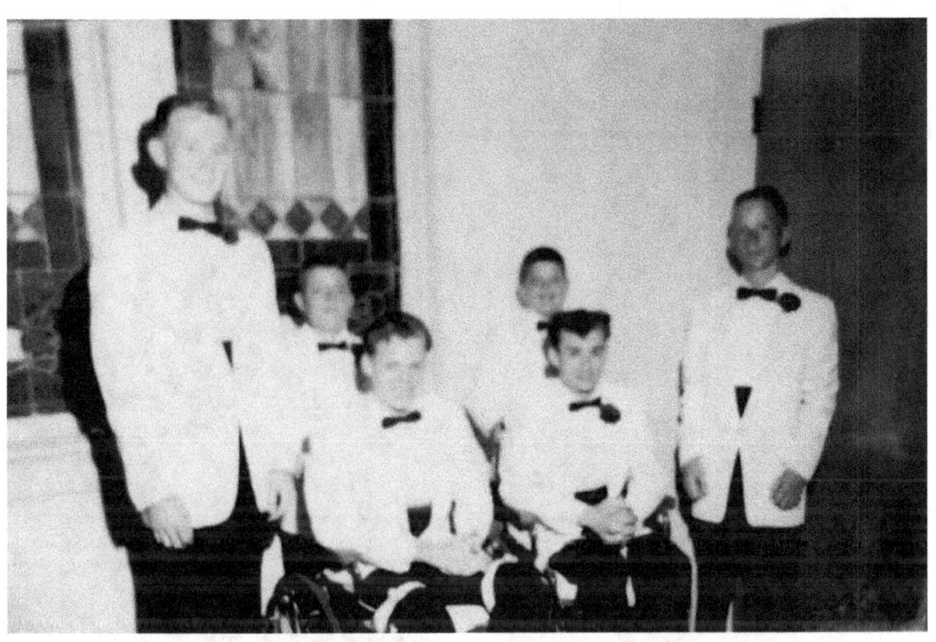

Jess and his dapper groomsmen.

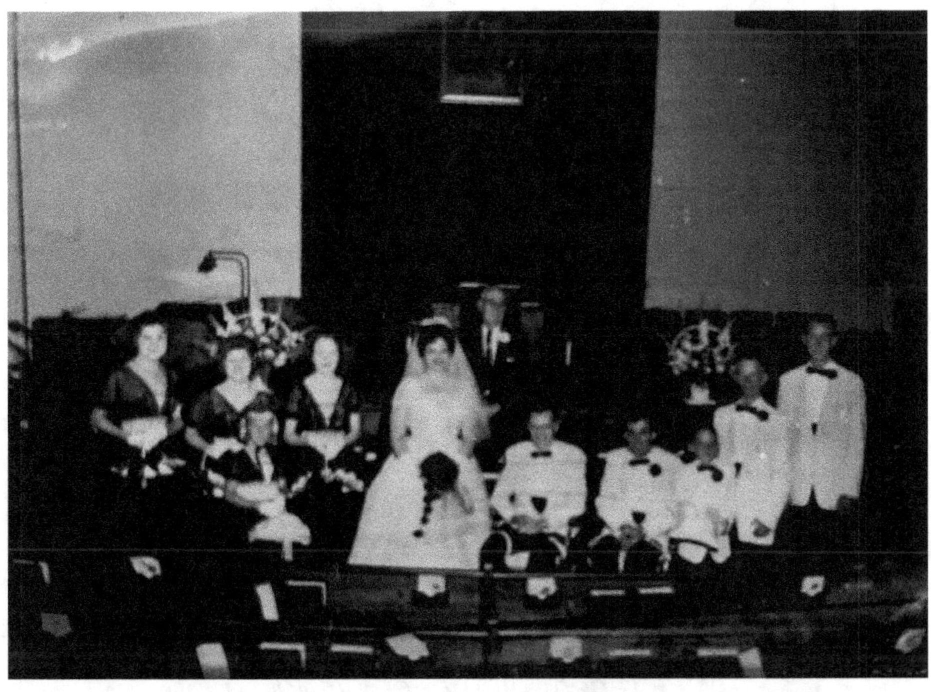

*Group photo of Lynda and Jess along with the bridesmaids
and groomsmen.*

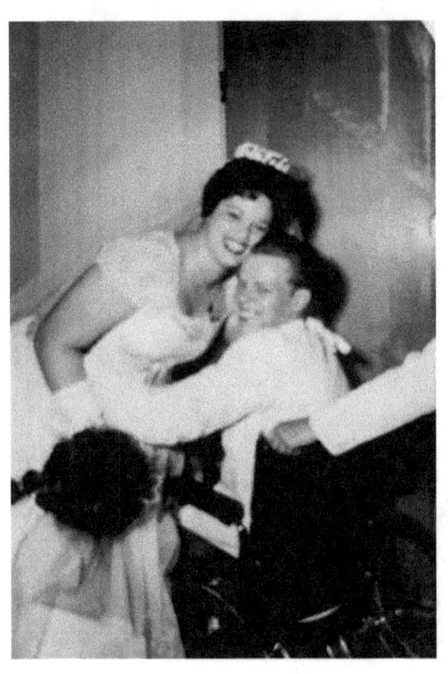

Shared, gleeful expressions.

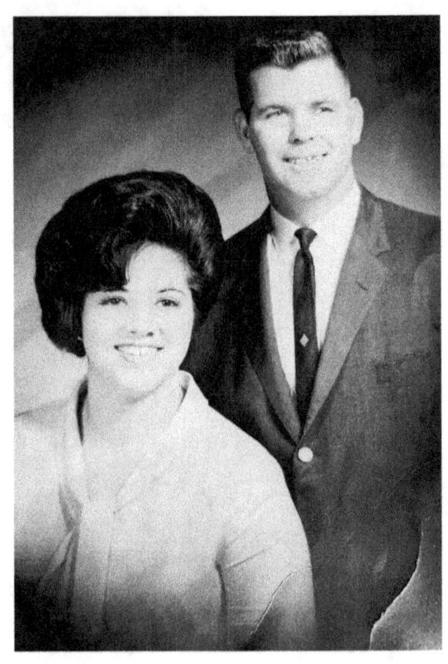

Portrait of Lynda and Carroll.

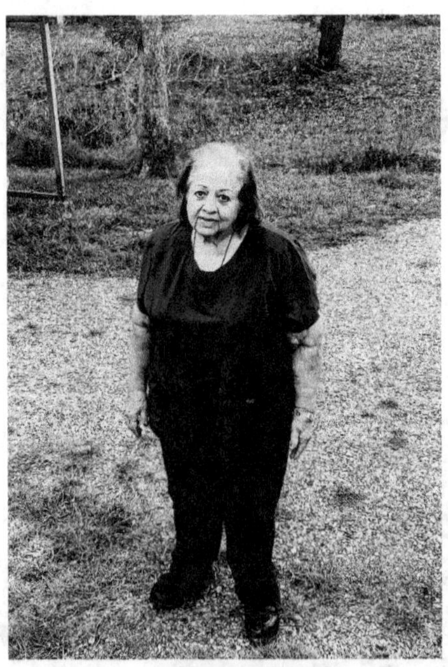

A recent picture of Lynda Johnson. A nurse of sixty-three years.

Common Abbreviations

- **AAROM** - *active assistive range of motion*
- **AAC** - *augmentative and alternative communication*
- **ABG** - arterial blood gas
- **AC** - *before meals*
- **A/C** - *assist control*
- **ADA Diet** - *American Diabetes Association Diet*
- **ADL** - *activities of daily living*
- **AFib** - *atrial fibrillation*
- **AKA** - *above-knee amputation*
- **ALS** - *amyotrophic lateral sclerosis*
- **AMA** - *against medical advice*
- **A&O** - *alert and oriented*
- **A/P** - *anterior-posterior*
- **AROM** - *active range of motion*
- **ASAP** - *as soon as possible*
- **ASD** - *autism spectrum disorder*
- **ASL** - *American Sign Language*
- **BID** - *twice a day*
- **BKA** - *below-knee amputation*
- **B/L** - *bilateral*
- **BLBS** - *bilateral breath sounds*
- **BMR** - *basal metabolism rate*
- **BP** - *blood pressure*
- **BR** - *bed rest*
- **bs** - *bowel sounds*
- **BS** - *breath sounds*
- **B/S** - *bedside*
- **BW** - *birth weight, body weight, blood work*
- **bx** - *biopsy*
- **c** - *with*
- **C** - *Celsius*

Common Abbreviations

- **C1 -** *first cervical vertebrae*
- **C2 -** *second cervical vertebrae*
- **CA** - *cardiac arrest*
- **ca** - *cancer, carcinoma*
- **CABG** - *coronary artery bypass graft*
- **CAD** - *coronary artery disease*
- **cal** - *calorie*
- **cath** - *catheter*
- **CBC** - *complete blood count*
- **cc** - *cubic centimeter*
- **CC** - *chief complaint*
- **CHF** - *congestive/chronic heart failure*
- **CCU** - *coronary care unit*
- **CHI** - *closed head injury*
- **cm** - *centimeter*
- **CN** - *cranial nerve*
- **CNA** - *certified nursing assistant*
- **CNS** - *central nervous system*
- **c/o** - *complains of*
- **COTA** - *certified occupational therapy assistant*
- **cont** - *continue(d)*
- **COPD** - *chronic obstructive pulmonary disease*
- **CP** - *cerebral palsy*
- **CPAP** - *continuous positive airway pressure*
- **CPR** - *cardiopulmonary resuscitation*
- **CRF** - *chronic renal failure*
- **CRNP** - *certified registered nurse practitioner*
- **CSF** - *cerebrospinal fluid*
- **CT** - *computerized tomography*
- **CV** - *cardiovascular*
- **CVA** - *cerebral vascular accident*

Common Abbreviations

- **CXR** - *chest X-ray*
- **d** - *day*
- **d/c** - *discontinue*
- **DC** - *discharge*
- **DM** - *diabetes mellitus*
- **DNK** - *do not know*
- **DNKA** - *did not keep appointment*
- **DNR** - *do not resuscitate*
- **DNT** - *did not test*
- **DOA** - *dead on arrival*
- **DOB** - *date of birth*
- **DOE** - *dyspnea on exertion*
- **d/t** - *due to*
- **Dx** - *diagnosis*
- **ECC, EKG** - *electrocardiogram*
- **ED** - *emergency department*
- **EEG** - *electroencephalogram*
- **EENT** - *eyes, ears, nose, throat*
- **EMG** - *electromyogram*
- **ENT** - *ears, nose, throat*
- **ER** - *emergency room*
- **ETOH** - *ethanol (alcohol)*
- **exam** - *examination*
- **ext** - *external, exterior*
- **F** - *Fahrenheit*
- **FH** - *family history*
- **fib** - *fibrillation*
- **fl** - *fluid*
- **f/u** - *follow-up*
- **FWB** - *full weight bearing*
- **Fx** - *fracture*

Common Abbreviations

- **GB** - *gallbladder*
- **GCS** - *Glasgow Coma Scale*
- **GE** - *gastroenterology*
- **GERD** - *gastroesophageal reflux disease*
- **G/E** - *gastroenteritis*
- **gen** - *general*
- **gest** -*gestation*
- **GI** - *gastrointestinal*
- **GNA** - *geriatric nurse assistant*
- **gluc** - *glucose*
- **GP** - *general practitioner*
- **GSW** - *gunshot wound*
- **GTT** - *glucose tolerance test*
- **GYN** - *gynecology*
- **h** - *hour*
- **H/A** - *headache*
- **HAV** - *hepatitis A virus*
- **Hb** - *hemoglobin*
- **HB** - *heart block*
- **HBP** - *high blood pressure*
- **HEENT** - *head, eyes, ears, nose, throat*
- **HEP** - *home exercise program*
- **H2O** - *water*
- **h/o** - *history of*
- **HOB** - *head of bed*
- **H&P** - *history and physical*
- **HR** - *heart rate*
- **HTN** - *hypertension*
- **HVD** - *hypertensive vascular disease*
- **Hx** - *history*
- **Hz** - *hertz (cycles/second)*

Common Abbreviations

- **ICCU** - *intensive coronary care unit*
- **ICP** - *intracranial pressure*
- **ICU** - *intensive care unit*
- **imp** - *impression*
- **incr** - *increase(d/ing)*
- **inf** - *infusion, inferior*
- **inspire** - *inspiration, inspiratory*
- **int** - *internal*
- **I&O** - *intake and output*
- **IPPB** - *intermittent positive pressure breathing*
- **irreg** - *irregular*
- **IV** - *intravenous(ly)*
- **J, jt** - *joint*
- **K** - *potassium, kidney*
- **L** - *left, liver, liter, lower, light, lumbar*
- **L2** - *second lumbar vertebrae*
- **L3** - *third lumbar vertebrae*
- **lab** - *laboratory*
- **lac** - *laceration*
- **lat** - *lateral*
- **LBW** - *low birth rate*
- **LE** - *lower extremities*
- **liq** - *liquid*
- **LOC** - *level of consciousness*
- **LP** - *lumbar puncture*
- **LPN** - *licensed practical nurse*
- **LUE** - *left upper extremity*
- **LVN** - *licensed vocational nurse*
- **Lx** - *larynx*
- **L&W** - *living and well*

Common Abbreviations

- **M** - *married, male, mother, murmur, meter, mass, molar*
- **max** - *maximum*
- **MBC** - *maximum breathing capacity*
- **MBSS** - *modified barium swallow study*
- **MCA** - *middle cerebral artery*
- **MD** - *muscular dystrophy*
- **mdnt** - *midnight*
- **med** - *medicine*
- **mets** - *metastasis*
- **MG** - *myasthenia gravis*
- **MI** - *myocardial infarction*
- **min** - *minute*
- **MICU** - *medical intensive care unit*
- **mod** - *moderate*
- **MRI** - *magnetic resonance imaging*
- **MRSA** - *methicillin-resistant Staphylococcus aureus*
- **mss** - *massage*
- **MVA** - *motor vehicle accident*
- **n** - *nerve*
- **Na** - *sodium*
- **NaCl** - *sodium chloride*
- **NAD** - *no abnormality detected, no apparent distress*
- **neg** - *negative*
- **neur** - *neurology*
- **NG** - *nasogastric*
- **NIC** - *neonatal intensive care*
- **NICU** - *neonatal intensive care unit*
- **NKA** - *no known allergies*
- **no** - *number*
- **NOS** - *not otherwise specified*
- **NPO** - *nothing by mouth*

Common Abbreviations

- **NSA** - *no specific abnormality*
- **NST** - *nonstress test*
- **N&V** - *nausea and vomiting*
- **NVD** - *nausea, vomiting, diarrhea*
- **N&W** - *normal and well*
- **NWB** - *non-weight bearing*
- **NYD** - *not yet diagnosed*
- **o** - *none, without*
- **O** - *oral*
- **O2** - *oxygen*
- **O2 cap** - *oxygen capacity*
- **O2 sat** - *oxygen saturation*
- **OA** - *osteoarthritis*
- **OB, OBG** - *obstetrics*
- **OB/GYN** - *obstetrics and gynecology*
- **Obs** - *observation*
- **OBS** - *organic brain syndrome*
- **ODD** - *oppositional defiant disorder*
- **O/E** - *on examination*
- **OH** - *occupational history*
- **OHD** - *organic heart disease*
- **oint** - *ointment*
- **OM** - *otitis media*
- **OME** - *otitis media with effusion*
- **OOB** - *out of bed*
- **Op** - *operation*
- **ot** - *ear*
- **Oto** - *otolaryngology*
- **OTC** - *over-the-counter (pharmaceuticals)*
- **OT** - *occupational therapy*
- **OR** - *operating room*

Common Abbreviations

- **PA** - *physician's assistant*
- **P&A** - *percussion and auscultation*
- **PACU** - *post-anesthesia care unit*
- **PAF** - *paroxysmal atrial fibrillation*
- **palp** - *palpate*
- **Path** - *pathology*
- **PA view** - *posterior-anterior view on X-ray*
- **p/c** - *after meals*
- **PD** - *Parkinson's disease*
- **pdr** - *powder*
- **PDN** - *private duty nurse*
- **PE** - *physical exam, pulmonary embolism*
- **Ped** - *pediatrics*
- **PEEP** - *positive end-expiratory pressure*
- **PEG** - *percutaneous endoscopic tomography*
- **PET** - *positron emission tomography*
- **PH** - *past history*
- **pharm** - *pharmacy*
- **PHYS** - *physical, physiology*
- **PI** - *present illness, pulmonary insufficiency*
- **PICU** - *pulmonary intensive care unit*
- **PID** - *pelvic inflammatory disease*
- **plts** - *platelets*
- **PM** - *afternoon, postmortem*
- **PMH** - *past medical history*
- **PMR** - *physical medicine and rehabilitation*
- **PN** - *practical nurse*
- **P&N** - *psychiatry and neurology*
- **PNA** - *pneumo, pneumonia*
- **PNI** - *peripheral nerve injury*

Common Abbreviations

- **PNX** - *pneumothorax*
- **po** - *by mouth*
- **pod** - *postoperative day*
- **pos** - *positive*
- **post** - *posterior*
- **POSTOP** - *postoperative*
- **pot** - *potassium*
- **PR** - *proctology*
- **pre-op** - *preoperative*
- **prep** - *prepare for*
- **prm** - *physical and rehabilitation medicine*
- **prn** - *as often as necessary, as needed*
- **prod** - *productive*
- **Prog** - *prognosis*
- **PROM** - *passive range of motion*
- **pron** - *pronator*
- **prosth** - *prosthesis*
- **PSH** - *past surgical history*
- **Psych** - *psychiatry*
- **pt** - *patient*
- **PT** - *physical therapy*
- **PTA** - *prior to admission*
- **PTA pulse** - *posterior tibial artery pulse*
- **PUD** - *peptic ulcer disease*
- **PVD** - *peripheral vascular disease*
- **PVT** - *previous trouble*
- **PWB%** - *partial weight bearing with percent*
- **PX** - *physical examination*
- **q** - *every*
- **qh** - *every hour*

Common Abbreviations

- **qid** - *four times a day*
- **qt** - *quart*
- **quad** - *quadriplegic*
- **R** - *right, rub, rectal temperature*
- **RA** - *rheumatoid arthritis, right atrium*
- **rad** - *radial*
- **ram** - *rapid alternating movements*
- **RAtx** - *radiation therapy*
- **RBC** - *red blood count*
- **RCA** - *right coronary artery*
- **RCU** - *respiratory care unit*
- **RD** - *respiratory distress*
- **RDS** - *respiratory distress syndrome*
- **RE** - *reconditioning exercise*
- **reg** - *regular*
- **rehab** - *rehabilitation*
- **resp** - *respiratory, respirations*
- **RF** - *rheumatic fever*
- **RLAS** - *Rancho Los Amigos Scale*
- **R to L&A** - *react to light and accommodation*
- **RLE** - *right lower extremity*
- **RN** - *registered nurse*
- **RND** - *radical neck dissection*
- **RO** - *rule out*
- **ROM** - *range of motion, rupture of membranes, right otitis media*
- **ROS** - *review of symptoms*
- **RT** - *radiation therapy, respiratory therapy*
- **RUE** - *right upper extremity*
- **RV** - *residual volume*
- **RW** - *rolling walker*

Common Abbreviations

- **Rx** - *prescription*
- **S** - *sensation, sensitive, serum*
- **Sa** - *saline*
- **sc** - *subcutaneous(ly)*
- **SCC** - *squamous cell carcinoma*
- **SCCA** - *squamous cell carcinoma antigen*
- **SCD** - *sudden cardiac death*
- **SCI** - *spinal cord injury*
- **schiz** - *schizophrenia*
- **SCU** - *special care unit*
- **sec** - *second*
- **Sens** - *sensory*
- **sep** - *separated*
- **SGA** - *small for gestational age*
- **SH** - *social history*
- **SI** - *stroke index*
- **sib** - *sibling*
- **SICU** - *surgical intensive care unit*
- **SIDS** - *sudden infant death syndrome*
- **skel** - *skeletal*
- **SL** - *under the tongue*
- **SLP** - *speech language pathologist*
- **sm** - *small*
- **SNF** - *skilled nursing facility*
- **SOAP** - *subjective, objective, assessment, plan*
- **SOB** - *shortness of breath*
- **S/P** - *status post*
- **sp cd** - *spinal cord*
- **spec** - *specimen*
- **sp fl** - *spinal fluid*
- **SP&H** - *speech and hearing*

Common Abbreviations

- **spin** - *spine, spinal*
- **spont** - *spontaneous*
- **s/s** - *signs and symptoms*
- **SS** - *social services*
- **ST** - *speech therapy*
- **stat** - *immediately*
- **STD** - *sexually transmitted disease*
- **subcut** - *subcutaneous*
- **sup** - *superior*
- **supin** - *supination*
- **surg** - *surgery, surgical*
- **Sx** - *symptoms*
- **sys** - *system*
- **syst** - *systolic*
- **T** - *temperature*
- **T&A** - *tonsillectomy and adenoidectomy*
- **tab** - *tablet*
- **TAH** - *total abdominal hysterectomy*
- **TB** - *tuberculosis*
- **TBI** - *traumatic brain injury*
- **temp** - *temperature*
- **THERAP** - *therapy, therapeutic*
- **THR** - *total hip replacement*
- **TIA** - *transient ischemic attack*
- **TKR** - *total knee replacement*
- **TNM** - *tumor, nodes, and metastases*
- **TO** - *telephone order*
- **TPN** - *total parenteral nutrition*
- **TPR** - *temperature, pulse, respiration*
- **tr** - *trace*
- **trach** - *tracheostomy*

Common Abbreviations

- **tsp** - *teaspoon*
- **Tx** - *treatment, therapy*
- **U/A** - *urinalysis*
- **UCD** - *usual childhood diseases*
- **Unilat** - *unilateral*
- **u/o** - *under observation*
- **Ur** - *urine*
- **URD** - *upper respiratory disease*
- **URI** - *upper respiratory infection*
- **Urol** - *urology*
- **US** - *ultrasound*
- **UTI** - *urinary tract infection*
- **V** - *vein*
- **VA** - *visual acuity*
- **vag** - *vagina*
- **VC** - *vital capacity*
- **VD** - *venereal disease*
- **vent** - *ventilator*
- **vert** - *vertical*
- **VF** - *ventricular fibrillation*
- **VFSS** - *videofluoroscopic swallowing study*
- **via** - *by way of*
- **vit** - *vitamin*
- **VN** - *visiting nurse*
- **VO** - *verbal order*
- **VS** - *vital signs*
- **wk** - *week*
- **W/C** - *wheelchair*
- **WBT** - *weight-bearing tolerance*
- **WFL** - *within functional limits*
- **w/n** - *within*

Common Abbreviations

- **WNL** - *within normal limits*
- **wt** - *weight*
- **w/u** - *workup*
- **x** - *times*
- **yo** - *years old*
- **yrs** - *years*

Tips & Advice for Student Nurses

Study Groups:
Meeting other students can help you retain information, fill in knowledge gaps, and motivate you to study. Plus, it lets you network with others who might benefit your career.

Create a Study Schedule:
A daily study schedule can help you stay on track with assignments and labs. A routine schedule also cultivates excellent habits you'll abide by in the workplace.

Know Your Learning Style:
If you've somehow found your way into nursing school without figuring out your own individual learning style, then there's no time like the present to learn. Understanding your learning style will save you time and spare you headaches.

Avoid Cramming:
Avoid cramming for exams and tests. Being proactive with your studies can help you avoid burnout, and as a result, you'll perform better.

Ask Questions:
Ask relevant questions to your mentors and/or superiors. Though it may initially seem daunting, these people are your best resource and lifeline. Remember, they've been where you are now. They understand.

Tips & Advice for Student Nurses

Practice Critical Thinking:
Critical thinking is a crucial skill for medical professionals. There's no better way to develop this skill than through continuous study and first-hand experience in school and the workplace.

Practice Self-Care:
Self-care can help you manage stress and promote safety and quality care. Remember, nurses are the backbone of the healthcare industry. If you can't adequately or effectively fulfill your duties, neither can your workplace. So remember to take time daily to love yourself and do something for yourself.

Prioritize Assignment:
Always prioritize assignments as they are given. This will help you manage your time in school and is a proactive habit you can implement in the workplace.

Don't Compare Yourself to Others:
Every person is unique. You have your own strengths and learning needs. Comparing yourself to others will never be beneficial. It will only put you and others down.

Take Care of Yourself:
You need to prioritize yourself. Period. It's okay to be selfish. Your physical and mental health are essential.

Tips & Advice for Current Nurses

Keep Learning:
New innovations and practices are constantly emerging in the medical field. It is imperative that you continually educate yourself. You never know when your educational knowledge can safeguard yourself, a coworker, or a patient.

Connect With Your Team:
All nurses should strive to work in unison regardless of preferences or personalities. You don't have to like each other or be friends outside of work, but you should never allow your personal feelings or opinions to overshadow your duty to your work team and purpose as a nurse.

Practice Self-Compassion:
In your occupation, there's always a chance that you'll have a rough day. You must remember that even though you had a 'bad day,' that does not make you a 'bad nurse.' It only proves that you are human like everyone else.

Develop Communication Skills:
Communicating effectively can help you inform, motivate, and lead others around you.

Stay Organized:
Sometimes, you have a tight schedule. Creating checklists, planning ahead, and delegating can prove helpful.

Tips & Advice for Current Nurses

Find A Mentor:
If possible, find and build a relationship with a nurse mentor. Doing this can accelerate your learning of various skills and help you avoid mistakes.

Prioritize Patient Care:
At the start of your shift, focus on the most urgent or critical needs. That way, you can be ahead of the curve, and essential actions aren't swept under the rug.

Practice Self-Care:
Nurses are exposed to the results of many horrors and evils in the world. The nursing occupation can interfere with your social and family life. You need some time to be yourself. To meditate and/or relax. Otherwise, you will be over-stressed and possibly be burned out.

Ask Questions:
Asking questions can help you know and understand the needs of your co-workers and patients. The action builds trust with others.

Don't Lose Yourself:
While on duty, you learn to put yourself and your personal feelings aside. Over time, it becomes very easy to forget that you're not only a nurse. Outside of work, there will be conversations, actions, and sounds that might cause you to go into nurse mode. Remember to have people and things that tether you back to who you are as a person.

Tips & Advice for Current Nurses

Safeguard Your Character & Dignity:
Unfortunately, there will always be politics and those who yearn for power in the workplace. That is why it's essential to always do your due diligence by keeping a detailed, accurate record of your patient and associated actions. Leave no room for questions or debate. This is important to safeguard yourself and your license.

The Nurse Never Leaves You:
Even after retirement, your nursing habits and experiences will likely never leave you. There will always be an accident, siren, or news caption that triggers a sense of anticipation for a patient you will never see. Though your selfless career has ended, in a moment of distress, you will yearn to help and assist. **Once a nurse, always a nurse.**

First Aid & Tell-Tale Signs

Burns:
Run fresh water over the burn for at least 20 minutes as soon as possible after the burn occurs.

Cuts & Scrapes:
Apply pure aloe vera gel to the wound to help it heal quickly and protect it from infection.

Blisters & Burns:
Apply antibiotic ointment to the wound as soon as possible after the injury to prevent infection and speed healing.

Fractures:
If you're trained in how to splint, apply a splint above and below the fracture site. Padding the splint can help reduce discomfort.

Pain:
Apply an ice pack or rub the area to relieve pain.

Cuts, Wounds, Skin Infections, and Itchy Areas:
Apply apple cider vinegar to soothe the skin and aid healing

Toothache:
If there are no other medical options, *you can place an aspirin on the achy tooth and keep it in place with your tongue. Over time, it will dissolve and temporarily soothe the ache.* ***However, doing this can damage the gums and other soft tissues in your mouth.***

First Aid & Tell-Tale Signs

Bleeding:
Apply pressure to the wound and pour a generous amount of black or cayenne pepper into the wound. The pepper will help stop the bleeding and seal the wound.

How to Tell If Someone Has a Broken Hip:
If someone's foot lays over flat on the floor, their hip is broken. Do not move this person if you are not medical personnel.

Cleaning:
Use an antiseptic agent to clean wounds and hands

Pain Relief:
Use acetaminophen, ibuprofen, or aspirin to relieve pain, fever, and headaches.

Sprains & Strains:
Use elastic wraps to wrap injuries to the wrist, ankle, knee, and elbow.

Heat Stress/Exhaustion:
Strive to remove yourself from the hot setting. Strive to slowly cool your body down. Sit upright and drink fluids with electrolytes to relieve symptoms. Watermelon juice works very well.

Shock:
If someone feels faint or is experiencing shortness of breath, lay them down with their head slightly lower than their trunk.

First Aid & Tell-Tale Signs

Nausea and Upset Stomach:
Ingesting ginger can help alleviate these symptoms. If you have difficulty ingesting raw ginger, try ginger tea or candied ginger.

Pain Relief:
Arnica cream can help relieve muscle aches, pains, and bruising
.

Irritated Skin:
Calendula can help skin irritations like eczema and diaper rash. Petroleum jelly can also keep skin moisturized and prevent chaffing.

Sleep:
Chamomile tea can help you relax in the evening. Allowing you to more easily fall to sleep.

Cold & Flu:
Hot liquids like tea and soup can help reduce mucus buildup and hydrate you.

Sore Throat:
You can gargle warm salt water to relieve this symptom. To step up the potency, add a little bit of turmeric to the warm salt water.

Diabetes:
If a person's breath smells like Juicy Fruit gum, they are probably diabetic.

First Aid & Tell-Tale Signs

Stomach Churning Smells:
To resist heinous smells, you must master breathing through your mouth rather than relying on your nose.

How to Make an Male External Catheter
I share this in honor of Jess, my first husband. These are the materials he used to construct the device:

1 Condom
1 Rubber Tube
1 Leg Bag

- *Grab the rubber tube and cut two thin pieces off the end. These thin pieces should be circular, like a rubber band.*
- Grab the condom and unroll it down the end of the rubber tube. The tip of the condom should touch the end of the tube.
- *Once the condom is in place, set 1 rubber band piece around the condom-covered tube. Set the rubber band about half an inch above the tip of the condom.*
- Tightly pull the remaining loose portion of the condom down towards its tip. Afterward, put the second rubber band piece over the overlapped condom next to the first rubber band.
- *With the second rubber band in place, cut the tip of the condom and the end of the tube off. This will make a hole for the person's urine to flow freely.*

First Aid & Tell-Tale Signs

- *Then firmly pull the opening of the condom over the male's penis. To prevent any leaks, secure the condom area with coban bandage strips. Ensure the bandage is not wrapped too tight so blood flow is not adversely affected.*
- *On the other end of the rubber tube, you connect and secure it to a leg bag. If this person intended to go outside, they could inconspicuously conceal this leg bag by laying it flat against their leg in their pants. It was not noticeable this way.*
- *If the leg bag needed to be emptied, there was a clip at the bottom of the bag that sealed its drain. After emptying it, you could roll the drain and clip it again.*

QR CODES

NAMI Hotline for Suicide Prevention

SAMHSA Helpline for Substance Abuse

National Problem Gambling Helpline

Health Insurance Marketplace

ANA Enterprise:
American Nurses Association

Honored Abilities Products